SLOW CARB
FOR LIFE

Published by ECW Press
2120 Queen Street East, Suite 200, Toronto, Ontario, Canada M4E 1E2

NATIONAL LIBRARY OF CANADA CATALOGUING IN PUBLICATION

Haakonson, Patricia, 1950–
Slow carb for life : the ultimate practical guide for low-carb living / Patricia Haakonson and
Harv Haakonson.

ISBN 1-55022-680-0

1. Complex carbohydrate diet. I. Haakonson, Harv, 1940– II. Title.

RM222.2.H33 2004   613.2'83

Editing: Joy Gugeler
Cover and Text Design: Tania Craan
Cover photo: Michael Tourigny
Typesetting: Mary Bowness
Printing: Webcom

This book is set in AGaramond.

The publication of *Slow Carb for Life* has been generously supported
by the Canada Council, the Ontario Arts Council, the Government
of Canada through the Book Publishing Industry
Development Program. **Canada**

DISTRIBUTION
CANADA: Jaguar Book Group, 100 Armstrong Avenue, Georgetown, ON, L7G 5S4
UNITED STATES: Independent Publishers Group, 814 North Franklin Street,
Chicago, Illinois 60610

PRINTED AND BOUND IN CANADA

ECW PRESS
ecwpress.com

SLOW CARB FOR LIFE

The Ultimate Practical Guide
to Low-Carb Living

PATRICIA HAAKONSON, B.SC.
HARV HAAKONSON, M.D.

ECW PRESS

Table of Contents

FOREWORD

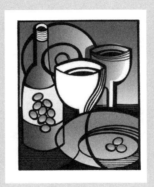

Foreword

Patricia's Story

In the fall of 1999, shortly after retirement, I began to ponder the new year and my upcoming 50th birthday (a monumental milestone). I wanted to finally lose the extra pounds I had accumulated over 30 years. Like many of you, I had tried a variety of different diets with limited success, but even if I lost weight I couldn't keep it off. Part of my problem was that I loved food! I loved to cook, I loved to bake, and I loved to eat.

Deciding to try a low-carb approach to diet was a decision I did not take lightly. At the time low-carb diets were receiving a lot of negative press, so I decided to try a modified approach and stick to it for two weeks. I was determined not to be "50 and fat!" My experience was both typical and unusual. During the two-week trial period, I noticed a number of dramatic changes in my health — all of which I attributed to a change in eating habits and food choices. I seemed to have more energy. I was not taking the afternoon naps that had become part of my routine, nor was I nodding off after dinner while trying to read or watch TV. I was surprised and delighted to discover that I was not hungry all the time, nor did I feel deprived. But the most life-changing result of the diet was that I no longer had symptoms of colitis (a digestive disease I had had since my late teens).

With the improvement in my health, and the desired weight loss, I am healthier today in my mid-50s than I was in my 20s. I have kept off the 40 pounds I lost for over four years, and I cannot imagine anything tempting me to return to my old habits. I continue to have energy all day long, the colitis has disappeared, and I am told I look 10 years younger. I still love to cook, bake, and eat, but I have a greater understanding of the foods I eat and their impact on my body. I eat differently, but without sacrificing flavor or my beloved desserts.

Frustrated with the lack of information about low-carb alternatives, and in particular the paucity of interesting low-carb recipes (remember, I still love food), my husband and I decided to write our own guide based on what we had learned.

If I was going to stick to this plan for the remainder of my life, I would need greater variety. The cookbooks available at the time not inspiring — so I set out to write my own. I was trying to develop low-carb recipes for our family when a friend suggested I might share them with other low carbers.

So, while I no longer think of myself as retired, I do think of myself as someone blessed with health, happiness, and a vocation that brings enormous satisfaction, especially when we hear from readers from all over the world. Imagine finding all that after 50!

Harv's Story

I came to the slow-carb life more reluctantly than Patricia. Although I was substantially above my ideal weight, I was physically active and had plenty of energy so saw no need to alter the way I ate. I hadn't decided to lose weight, but after watching the dramatic changes in Patricia's life and witnessing her new outlook, I began to give some serious thought to trying this myself. Though Patricia was on a low-carb diet, she had continued cooking me potatoes and rice. After seeing her energy increase and the end of her debilitating colitis symptoms, I decided to forgo the potatoes and the bread and give it a try.

Perhaps my medical training made me skeptical; how could a simple shift in eating habits control my weight? Over a period of a few months I lost 38 pounds and returned to my ideal weight, which I had not been able to maintain since I was an intern. I felt great! I too experienced an increase in energy. I trained for and ran the Boston Marathon in 2001, only the second marathon in my life, in a very respectable 3:30:45. I began to do some serious reading in medical journals and checked other sources to better understand why and how this plan garnered such positive results. I re-educated myself. I was pleasantly surprised when my own family doctor informed me that both my cholesterol and my blood pressure were lower than normal. He remarked, "Harv, what have you done? You seem to have found the fountain of youth!"

I continue to be amazed by how easy it is to maintain this lifestyle while eating as well as we do (I am always happy to test Patricia's new recipes). I have maintained my ideal weight for over four years, and like Patricia, cannot imagine going back to my old habits. As nutritionists try to better understand diet and its impact on health, I learn with them. I am humbled by the response to our previous books and feel privileged to have the opportunity to meet so many readers either in person, over radio and TV airwaves, or in cyberspace.

Because we've personally embarked upon the journey you are considering, each approaching the slow-carb lifestyle from slightly different perspectives and viewpoints, we decided to include our individual stories and "before" photos to reassure you we are speaking from experience.

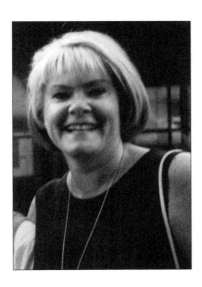 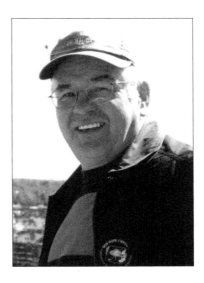

OVERVIEW OF THE SLOW-CARB PROGRAM

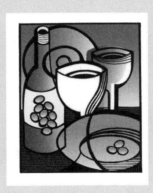

Overview of the Slow-Carb Program

Slow Carb for Life is based on the practice of choosing to eat good carbohydrates that convert slowly into blood sugar rather than arbitrarily reducing all carbohydrates. These slow carbs will help you realize the weight loss and dramatically improved health that typical diets can't deliver over the long term. This is not a diet, but rather a permanent and healthy lifestyle change that will inspire you to eat this way for health, as well as for life.

The slow carb approach offers a balanced diet of nutritious food in normal-sized portions. It does not require purchasing specialized meals, but it does require a new attitude toward food. Changing your lifelong eating habits will result in a slimmer, trimmer physique; increased energy and well-being; reduced bad cholesterol and increased good cholesterol; and decreased blood pressure.

Slow Carb for Life is the result of more than four years of personal trial and error while experimenting with a low-carb lifestyle. During this period we have researched, read, analyzed, and digested an enormous amount of material related to low-carbohydrate and other kinds of diets, the insulin mechanism, nutrition, food preparation, and exercise. We published *Easy Low-Carb Cooking* in 2001 and *Easy Low-Carb Living* in 2002. We have investigated and responded to literally thousands of Web site questions: What is a slow carb? How does a slow carb plan work? How is this approach different from other low-carb diets? Will it help me lose weight? Will it improve my general health? Is it difficult to put into practice? Do I really have to eat this way for life?

This book will share our findings and include some of those readers' (people of every age and walk of life) comments, suggestions, testimonials, and stories to instruct and inspire you. The comments are unsolicited feedback from individuals who have succeeded in their quest for weight loss and improved health. In addition to our successes and failures, and lessons we learned from our mistakes, these e-mails allowed us to fine-tune our recommendations and develop creative solutions to your problems as we consider situations beyond our own experience. This has also allowed us to identify why some people have difficulties following this program, to revisit topics that require further explanation, and to make revisions, adaptations, and changes. We have been impressed by the experiences our readers have shared with us, and we hope that their successes will in turn inspire you.

The slow carb approach and our guidelines are based on hard science and sound research combined with first-hand experience and valuable feedback. Simple explanations of complicated scientific discoveries and principles make a complex subject easier to understand; we have attempted to provide you with sufficient information and tools to be your own advisor. After learning how to assess your food options, you will find over 150 simple-to-prepare and delicious low-carb recipes to help make eating this way an enjoyable and fulfilling experience.

Because we want you to be successful in achieving your goals, we share all of our own strategies for success and endeavor to eliminate most of the guesswork, from helpful hints about how to eat slow-carb when you go out to dinner to fail-safe plans for when you go on vacation. You will find menu planning for weight loss, for maintenance, for adolescents, and for entertaining. We also provide a Food Diary, as well as a Carb Counter, to help you track your food intake and exercise. We explain in detail how to use these tools to the best advantage and where to go for low-carb products, resources, and the answers to your questions.

Together we lost more than 80 pounds while following this moderate low-carb approach. We have been able to maintain this weight loss for over four years, with no sense of deprivation or the punishment of being "on a diet." During this period we have drawn many conclusions about what works well and what is less effective, what to do about stalled weight loss, and how to find your individual carb level for weight maintenance. We believe that we are in the midst of a diet revolution that will medically prove a slow-carb lifestyle to be the accepted heart-healthy alternative to low-fat diets. We also believe that extremely low-carb plans are unnecessary for most people; they are very difficult to maintain and can feel punishing, due in part to the elimination of all fruits. A moderate slow carb plan with a balanced approach to nutrition is much easier to maintain, as our readers have confirmed.

In the following chapter we discuss how the body converts or metabolizes carbohydrates into blood sugar through the insulin mechanism. Some of the blood sugar is readily available as energy for the body's use, some is converted into fat for deposit in fat cells, and some becomes blood fats that increase our risk of heart disease. Carbs that turn quickly to blood sugar — breads, potatoes, white rice, most pasta, pastry products, and sugar — have a high GI, and consumption of large quantities of these foods is likely to lead to obesity, high blood fats (cholesterol and triglycerides), high blood pressure, insulin resistance, diabetes, and periods of low energy.

When we eat any carbohydrates, a basic component of food (like protein and fat), they turn to blood sugar to provide energy for the body. Almost all foods have some carbohydrates, including fruits, vegetables, nuts and seeds, dairy products, eggs, grains, and grain products. The Glycemic Index (GI) is a measurement that scientists have developed to express how quickly or slowly a certain food turns to blood sugar. Many refined carbohydrates, such as white breads, bagels, pasta, and most baked goods, turn to blood sugar very quickly and therefore have a high GI. High GI foods cause an immediate spike in our blood sugar that alerts the pancreas to produce insulin. Because most North American diets have been loaded with carbohydrates over the past 30 years, our pancreas overproduces insulin, causing a precipitous drop in blood sugar. This type of eating causes a cycle of blood sugar spikes and lows that produce weight gain (caused by the conversion of the blood sugar to fat for storage), mood swings, and feelings of lethargy and drowsiness after eating. The blood sugar low may also produce hunger pangs that demand another sugar hit. This spiraling cycle is self-perpetuating and very harmful.

We can avoid all these negative effects simply by choosing to eat complex low glycemic carbohydrates such as fruits, vegetables, whole grains, nuts, and seeds, which turn to blood sugar more slowly, have a low GI, and allow you to avoid the blood sugar highs and lows that overload your pancreas (a problem that can lead to Type II Diabetes) and lead to mood swings, energy dips, or the hunger pangs associated with the blood sugar swings. Carbs with a low GI allow us to control our weight and keep our cholesterol, triglycerides, and blood pressure low. Furthermore, foods that have high fiber content slow the absorption of carbohydrates and reduce net carbohydrate content.

Common low GI carbohydrates include vegetables like broccoli, cauliflower, zucchini, lettuce, spinach, cucumber, and cabbage. The low GI fruits include strawberries, raspberries, blueberries, blackberries, kiwi, pineapple, peaches, and watermelon. We provide an extensive list of slow carb foods as well as guidelines to help you make good food choices. Once you have achieved your ideal weight, you will learn to maintain it by increasing your slow carb intake to the level you determine is appropriate.

Slow Carb for Life is not protein loaded, as are some other low-carb diets, but rather a balance of slow carb foods, good fats, and protein that achieves health benefits and weight control. We recommend normal protein portions with meals and snacks to maintain consistent blood sugar levels and energy all day long. We also suggest lots of vegetables to fill you up, fruit, even during the weight loss period, and three normal-sized meals and two or three snacks every day.

Slow Carb for Life, like all low-carb programs, is based on the principles of metabolism, blood sugar conversion, and the insulin mechanism, but it is very different in its method of applying these scientific principles to your daily living. Our recommendations are not as extreme as other low-carb diets; we do not recommend restricting your carb intake level to 20 grams or less a day to lose weight, nor do we recommend "reward meals" that allow you to splurge and eat as many carbs as you want as long as the meal is eaten within certain time constraints. We also don't think it is wise to follow a low-carb plan for a short period in order to lose weight and then go back to old eating patterns. This is a new way of eating — for life.

Choosing to live a low-carb lifestyle and following the recommendations that are the basis for *Slow Carb for Life* requires fundamental shifts in your thinking when it comes to food shopping and preparation, re-education about certain foods, and carefully planning meals. There are many imaginative ways to vary meals and reintroduce certain foods into your diet (such as eggs, cream, and good fats), without fear of harmful effects and low-carb prepared or pre-packaged foods are available in most grocery and health food stores. Your choices and meal preparation can be quick and easy, especially as there are a growing number of stores and

Web sites dedicated to low-carb products.

Our strategies for success help make this way of eating flexible and easy. You will be able to: eat in restaurants, at fast food outlets, and in the homes of your friends; and fully enjoy the holidays, go on vacation, and do all the things you want to do while eating a healthy diet that allows you to feel energetic and healthy.

Here is a snapshot *Slow Carb for Life* to do list to ensure you enjoy the same success that has benefited thousands of our readers.

Eat Slow Carbs: Choose carbohydrates with a low GI that will convert to blood sugar more slowly so that you enjoy high levels of energy all day and avoid the negative impact of the blood sugar highs and lows.

Keep a Food Diary: Some of our readers have difficulty losing weight but aren't able to identify why because they do not keep a Food Diary. A daily record of what foods you consume, and how many carbs you eat, is an essential step in re-educating yourself. It is vitally important to have this record in order to analyze fluctuations in your progress.

Weigh-in Weekly: It is rare for a weight loss plan to go exactly as you intend. Remember you are learning new ways to eat, so you are bound to make the occasional error in the beginning. Weigh-ins will help you make adjustments if the pounds are not coming off.

Exercise: Any healthy lifestyle must include regular exercise. It isn't necessary to be a marathon runner, or to bench-press 250 pounds, to be healthy. It is essential to exercise at least four times a week. The most universally available and inexpensive exercise is walking.

Keep Meals Simple: This plan does not require special ingredients or expensive or hard-to-find prepared foods. Preparation times are short, and widely available ingredients and a variety of recipes make our plan easy to integrate into your lifestyle.

Stick to the Plan When Eating Out: Of course you can control your food and eat this way at home, but you must also be able to eat this way at work or on the road. The average North American family eats out at least once a week. Our meal plans and strategies offer the kind of flexibility you need to stay on your program when you dine out or eat a friend's.

Listen to Your Body: Nobody wants to hear that they can never eat a favorite food again, so it is important that this lifestyle can accommodate the occasional splurge. Furthermore, each of us will require a different carb intake to maintain our ideal weight. The recommendations in our plan will accommodate these differences and preferences.

Read Labels: Become a knowledgeable consumer and diligent reader of labels when you do your shopping, whether for groceries or special low-carb foods or snacks.

Change Your Lifestyle: In order for you to be successful, it is essential to make the mental shift to thinking of this as a lifestyle, a permanent change. You have chosen to eat differently for the rest of your life. This is not a diet.

Following these principles has enabled thousands of our readers to adopt this way of eating to control their weight and improve their health.

Joel: Sidney, British Columbia

Hello Harv and Patricia,

I thought you might be interested in hearing about my successes with the help of your two books. I lost the first 20 pounds before Christmas and now I am starting the second 20-pound phase of my weight loss. It is easy; I feel the weight melting off! I don't feel deprived and I sure don't miss the white stuff — the potatoes, bread, rice, or pasta. I get lots of positive comments about my weight loss and I give instant credit to your sensible low-carbohydrate eating plan.

This is my weight loss story. With an early retirement at 55, I focused on finally getting fit, since a busy career in health care administration had left little time to care for myself. I knew the benefits of good health, but I didn't have the energy to allocate to my own health. So having thought through some specific new year's resolutions about better lifestyle choices, and along with my newly retired husband, we headed off to the weight room at the Panorama Recreation Center in Sidney. We made it a five-days-a-week, one-and-a-half-hour morning commitment. With the help of our kinesiologist, Susan, we had individualized workout programs designed for our age and ability — cardiovascular workouts, weight lifting, and mat work. After seven months I was feeling stronger, fitter, more flexible, but still carrying the same weight as when I started. I was really discouraged! I was easily 50 pounds overweight and I was working too hard not to be seeing better results! My husband was losing weight with no difficulty.

Was it related to hormones, I wondered? So I turned to some references, in particular, *The Wisdom of Menopause* by Christiane Northup, MD. I also attended a lecture by Pamela Peakes, MD. Both sources suggested, especially during menopause, lowering carbohydrates and sugars and increasing exercise.

Coincidentally I spotted your two books on a friend's coffee table and was immediately drawn to the simplicity of the format. The next day I located the books at Tanners Bookstore in Sidney. It was my plan to read them during the summer and once I had digested them (so to speak) I would start making changes to my eating in September. That all changed when I read them. I was ready to start, then and there.

I began by using the daily food diary and following the meal plans in the book. The recipes are easy to follow and very tasty. I frequently use them when entertaining. I had a five-pound weight loss the first week and then a steady and gradual loss up to Christmas. Then I gave myself permission to enjoy the season with a few more carbs than recommended! However, I started back on the low carbs right after Christmas and by my first weigh-in on January 6 I was at my pre-Christmas weight. I started toward my second goal to lose another 20 pounds. I've tried a lot of strategies to lose weight over the years, but I can honestly say this method is the easiest and most effective. Thank you for these great books — they are a staple in my kitchen.

UNDERSTANDING CARBOHYDRATES

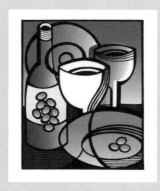

Understanding Carbohydrates

If you listen to a panel of experts discuss diets, you will likely find their recommendations confusing and contradictory. With a new diet fad, miracle weight loss pill, supplement program, or book on the market every day, how do we make sense of it all without more than a general knowledge of nutrition, anatomy, and physiology?

Since writing our first book, *Easy Low-Carb Living*, the proliferation of conflicting information about low-carb diets has continued, yet there have also been many important clinical studies that support low-carb eating for weight loss and its other important health benefits. We have continued to study this field and feel there is a sufficient volume of new material to revise many of our original recommendations. This is not a scientific textbook expected to satisfy the scientific reader; it is designed as a basic text for anyone concerned about weight and health. Because you are at least considering adopting a slow-carb lifestyle (why else would you be reading this book?), it is important you understand the mechanism that could make weight loss, and weight control, easier than you imagined.

The lifestyle we have developed does not follow what is traditionally known as a low-carb diet; we do not protein load, we are very conscious to limit the amount of saturated fat we eat, we have intentionally increased the amount of good fat we consume, and we believe in the importance of a nutritionally balanced plan that includes fruit. Certainly our carbohydrate intake is reduced, but more importantly the carbohydrates are slow to convert to blood sugar.

The human body is wonderfully complex. In order to perform any of its many functions, it needs energy from food and drink to fuel its bodily functions. There are only three types of food energy available to the body: carbohydrates, fats, and proteins. For as long as we can remember we have been urged by medical and nutritional experts to avoid fat at all costs. Carbohydrates have been accepted, even promoted, as the mainstay of our diet. It turns out our experts have been wrong on both counts. Fats aren't bad, at least not all bad, and carbohydrates aren't all good, at least not in the form and quantities we have become accustomed to eating.

When the body receives food, it has to choose which type of fuel to burn first — carbohydrate, fat, or protein. The body will always follow the path of least resistance and the fuel easiest to burn is carbohydrate. You likely know this from your own experience. When you need quick energy, if you are like most North Americans, you eat a chocolate bar or a bag of chips, or drink a soda. In each case the fuel you consumed was carbohydrate that converted quickly to blood sugar. As soon as this happens, the pancreas is stimulated to release a surge of insulin to force the sugar (glucose) into muscle, liver, and fat cells. The sugar can then be used for immediate energy (muscles), or stored for the short term (liver) or long-term (body fat).

In the last 30 years the proportion of our food that is carbohydrate has increased substantially. This is clear by comparing the consumption of refined sugar (in all forms) and grain. Montignac, in his book *Eat Yourself Slim*, points out that in the late 1700s the French consumed less than two pounds of sugar per person per year. By 1880 it was 17 pounds a year, at the turn of the century it was up to 37 pounds, and today it is 83 pounds per person per year. The Center for Science in the Public Interest in the U.S. reports, "Sugar consumption has been going through the roof. It has increased by 28 percent since 1983, fueling soaring obesity rates and other health problems. It's vital that the FDA require labels that would enable consumers to monitor — and reduce — their sugar intake." The average North American consumes an astonishing 130 pounds of sugar per person per year; though some sources say it is closer to 158 pounds. And sugar isn't the only culprit. The U.S. Department of Agriculture reports that in 1970 the average North American ate 135 pounds of grain. In 1997 that figure was 200 pounds.

Comparing Sample Carbohydrate Diets

It is revealing to compare the carbohydrate content of a typical North American diet with generic sample diets that contain the carb levels we recommend for weight loss or maintenance. The following three daily meal plans allow you to make that comparison.

Sample Typical North American Diet

		Grams of Carb	Fiber	Net Carb
Breakfast	1 cup orange juice	29	0	29
	1 cup raisin bran, sugar, 1/2 cup skim milk	75	8	67
	coffee with 1 teaspoon cream	0.5	0	0.5
10:00 a.m.	carrot muffin	30	2	28
	coffee with 1 teaspoon cream	0.5	0	0.5
Noon	turkey sandwich	49	7	42
	1 oz potato chips	21	0.7	20.3
	Coca-Cola	39	0	39
3:00 p.m.	granola bar — blueberry	35	3	32
	Coca-Cola	39	0	39
Dinner	grilled chicken breast	0	0	0
	baked potato with butter	51	4.8	46.2
	corn niblets	13	1	12
	dinner roll with butter	13	0	13
	2 chocolate chip cookies	30	2	28
	tea	0	0	0
9:00 p.m.	2 cookies	30	2	28
	tea	0	0	0
Total		455	30.5	424.5

Sample Slow-Carb Weight Loss Daily Meal Plan

		Net Grams of Carb
Breakfast	2 scrambled eggs	1.2
	2 strips of bacon	0
	coffee with cream	0.5
10:00 a.m.	Walnut Flax Muffin	2.4
	decaf coffee with cream	0.5
Noon	Chicken Salad	2.4
	1/2 cup coleslaw	4.2
	1/2 cup strawberries	3.6
3:00 p.m.	2 celery sticks, 2 tablespoons cream cheese	1.6
Dinner	broiled chicken breast	0
	1/2 cup steamed cauliflower	0.8
	1/2 cup steamed asparagus	1.9
	green salad with dressing	4.9
	1/2 cup raspberries	2.9
9:00 p.m.	sugar-free Jell-O	0
Total Carbohydrate Intake		26.9

Sample Slow-Carb Maintenance Daily Meal Plan

		Net Grams of Carb
Breakfast	1/2 cup All Bran Extra Fiber,	7.0
	1/4 cup light cream	1.0
	1/2 cup strawberries	3.6
	coffee with cream	0.5
10:00 a.m.	slice of Citrus Low-Carb Bar	4.4
	decaf coffee with cream	0.5
Noon	Mushroom and Spinach Frittata	3.1
	Marinated Veggies	6.8
3:00 p.m.	Walnut Flax Muffin	2.4
Dinner	roast chicken breast	0.0
	Creamy Garlic Cauliflower	3.0
	Grilled Zucchini	2.0
	Greens with Pecans & Blue Cheese	2.9
	Crème Brûlée	4.1
9:00 p.m.	sugar-free Jell-O	0.0
Total Carbohydrate Intake		41.3

In order to digest the high quantities of carbohydrates the typical North American diet contains, our body has become accustomed to releasing large amounts of insulin. If you eat a high carbohydrate meal consisting of a dinner roll, a baked potato, some carrots and peas, a piece of chocolate cake for dessert, and a teaspoon of sugar in your tea, your pancreas is going to release insulin, and lots of it. The insulin does its job, in fact probably overdoes it, because the pancreas can't be precise about how many carbohydrates have been consumed. Consequently, the insulin pushes more sugar into the muscle, liver, and fat cells than is ideal, lowering your blood sugar so that you feel lethargic, less mentally alert, and hungry. Your body's defense mechanism is to boost the blood sugar again so it prompts you to eat more carbohydrates to relieve your symptoms. The long-term effect of this cycle (too much carbohydrate followed by too much insulin) is that the body becomes less responsive to insulin or develops "insulin resistance" that causes the pancreas to produce even more insulin to get the job done. A permanently high insulin level is called "hyperinsulinism."

There are two other common medical conditions (they often go together) that are apt to result from this vicious cycle. Firstly, the high demand on the pancreas to produce insulin may wear it out and cause diabetes. Secondly, because the insulin is not being effective in converting the blood glucose into energy, it stores more and more of it as fat, which results in obesity. Studies have shown that both obese and diabetic individuals are often extremely unresponsive to insulin.

If you read extensively about diets and dieting, you may also know about Syndrome X. The medical community defines a condition as a syndrome when several medical conditions coexist, but there isn't an explanation as to why. Syndrome X is a cluster of metabolic disorders that include insulin resistance, obesity, blood fat abnormalities, glucose intolerance (diabetes), and high blood pressure. Syndrome X doesn't mean all of these conditions are always present, but some of them often occur simultaneously. Some scientists believe high carbohydrate intake creates abnormalities in the insulin mechanism, which contribute to the syndrome. By controlling carbohydrate intake those who might have the syndrome can correct some or all of these metabolic disorders.

Glycemic Index

Recent research indicates that carbohydrates are converted into sugar in the blood at varying rates. Some carbohydrates make blood sugar quickly, others much more slowly. Dr. David Jenkins, a researcher at the University of Toronto, developed a means of classifying foods according to how quickly they are broken down into sugar and absorbed into the bloodstream. This rating system is called the Glycemic Index (GI). Foods with a high GI become sugar so quickly that the ensuing insulin release is very damaging. The alternative, choosing carbohydrates with a low GI, results in a more sustained absorption into the bloodstream, which avoids a sudden insulin high. These are the slow-carb foods that are the core of our eating plan. If you make the effort to become familiar with the GI of foods you eat — carbs with a GI of 50 or less and whole or unrefined foods are best-you can make wiser decisions. We have taken much of the guesswork out of the decision making for you by providing lists of slow-carb foods in the Carbohydrate Counter at the end of this book.

Glycemic Load

Following the development of the GI, researchers at Harvard identified an even more accurate system known as the Glycemic Load (GL). This classification is based on multiplying the amount of carbohydrate (number of grams) in a normal serving of a food by the GI and dividing by 100, a complicated method that to be completely accurate has to be calculated in a clinical setting.

$$\frac{\text{grams of carb x GI}}{100} = GL$$

This level of accuracy isn't realistic in everyday living, nor is it essential if we merely want an indication of which carbohydrates are healthiest. Our Carbohydrate Counter gives you an easy reference for the number of grams of carbohydrate (in a normal serving) in many common foods. We have included the GI and calculated the GL where data is available. Familiarity with the GL of a food enables you to choose items that have the least insulin stimulating effect, a GL of 10 or less.

In order to keep it simple and successful, count the grams of carb and stay within your target amount each day. For example, an apple and a small boiled potato each have about 20 grams of carb, but an apple has a GI of 40 whereas the potato has a GI of 90. They have very different effects on your weight management and your health. The difference between the choices is most accurately, and most dramatically, demonstrated by calculating the GL. The apple, at 20 grams of carb and a GI of 40, has a GL of 8. The poor old potato on the other hand, with 20 grams of carb but with a GI of 90, has a GL of 18. The apple is within the guidelines we previously suggested, with a GI under 50 and a GL less than 10. Knowing how to use these additional tools gives you a much greater range of options. Don't worry if you prefer not to struggle with the formula; if you follow our guidelines and meal plans, we have done the calculations for you.

Net Carbs

Many packagers of low-carb foods (especially protein bars) use the term "net carbs" or "effective carb content." These manufacturers prefer to advertise as few carbs as possible in order to sell their products. In the past, manufacturers simply didn't include the carbs contained in fiber, sugar alcohols (like maltitol), or glycerine on the labeling. Most people don't absorb these ingredients, therefore they don't have an impact on blood sugar. Recently the U.S. FDA has legislated that all of these ingredients must be included in the total carb count. As a result, manufacturers now provide the net carb count as well as the total carbs in their product. We recommend that you only count the net carbs in your daily carb intake, as the remainder of the carbs made up of the fiber, maltitol, and glycerine don't normally get absorbed by your digestive system. It is unwise to eat more than one commercial low-carb bar per day since too much sugar alcohol and glycerine can cause digestive upset. Because some people absorb these ingredients, eating too many of these products can cause weight loss to stall. An alternative to these low-carb bars are the homemade protein bars found in the Recipe section.

Dietary Fiber

More and more low-carb foods are marketed by mentioning only the *net* carb content of the product. Drs. Michael and Mary Eades, in their book *The Protein Power Lifeplan*, present a related concept known as "effective carbohydrate content (ECC)." Their theory is that fiber, though it is a carbohydrate, is so complex that the body's digestive system cannot break it down into sugar to be absorbed in the blood. This means fiber does not stimulate the release of insulin and therefore does not contribute to the negative health effects we associate with high carbohydrate intake. Drs. Eades recommend that the fiber portion of food be left out of our daily carbohydrate calculation. This refinement can make a significant difference with some foods, though it does make your carb counting a little more complicated. For example, Kellogg's All Bran with Extra Fiber has a carb count of 20 grams, but 13 grams of that is dietary fiber that doesn't get absorbed so doesn't need to be counted in your daily total. The net carb count is then really seven grams. All our recipes include the fiber content in the nutrition calculation and calculate net carbs for your convenience.

The choice to live slow-carb avoids high insulin levels that may have other unhealthy effects, including

- salt and water retention, both of which contribute to high blood pres sure and obesity
- arteries that are more responsive to adrenaline, which aggravates high blood pressure
- high levels of triglycerides, blood fats involved in hardening of the arteries
- high levels of bad LDL cholesterol
- low levels of good HDL cholesterol
- sleep disorders.

It is important to remember that insulin isn't the enemy; it is just a hormone that deals with the poor choices we make when we eat. It is even more important to remember that if we eliminate those excesses and make better choices, we will reduce, or eliminate, the negative effects associated with insulin. Now that you understand how carbohydrates affect our ability to control our weight and maintain our health, it is time to turn our attention to the fats in our diet.

Glenda: Glace Bay, Nova Scotia

I had to write and say thanks! I bought your books and lost 31 pounds in three months following your "diet." I have gone from a (tight) size 16, to a very comfortable size 12 and my goal was to get into a 14! I just turned 50 in January and I last wore a size 12 in high school. I feel better now than I ever did, and everyone tells me I look great! Over the years, I tried every diet — Weight Watchers, Slim Fast, low fat, etc. Following your low-carb suggestions (I hate to use the word diet!) was so incredibly easy. I was someone who ate pasta perhaps five times a week and loved my breads and rice, but I don't miss them at all after going low-carb. Thank you both so very much!

UNDERSTANDING FATS

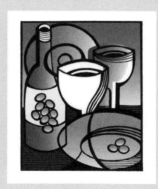

Understanding Fats

Until recently you could be forgiven for thinking that being overweight was simply the result of eating too much. We have been taught to believe that weight control is simply a matter of balancing calories in with calories out. But if it is that simple, why are more than half of North Americans overweight? One in every five is obese, that is, more than 20 percent above ideal body weight (Willett, p. 56). Drs. Michael and Mary Eades, authors of *The Protein Power Lifeplan*, believe that "74 percent of adult Americans are overweight to some degree" (p. 32). The U.S. Centers for Disease Control predict that if present trends continue, more than 50 percent of the U.S. population will be obese by 2010. The statistics are alarming and the health risks include, but are not limited to, heart disease, Type II Diabetes, stroke, high blood pressure, high cholesterol, and high triglycerides. Recent estimates suggest health costs for U.S. weight-related diseases has reached $3.5 billion annually.

Dr. Diana Schwarzbein, in her book *The Schwarzbein Principle II — The Transition*, says, "eating too many calories is not the reason people become fat, and counting calories will never make a person thin" (p. 16). One of the myths she debunks is that weight is related to caloric input versus caloric output. In her view, "Calories do not determine your body composition (weight); your hormones do. This is because your hormones determine your current metabolism. Restricting your calories to lose weight leads to a low insulin (hormone) effect that will eventually destroy your metabolism. Do not make the mistake of counting calories. Eat balanced meals to keep your hormones balanced and your metabolism working efficiently" (p. 108).

Why Have Low Fat Diets Failed?

Eating too many calories contributes to being overweight, and fat can make up a lot of those calories, but these are not the principal villains. Carbohydrate intake and the hyperinsulinism it causes is the real culprit. When we read the labels on low-fat foods we find added sugar and other sugar products that dramatically increase the carb content. So, while we thought we were eating the correct foods, we were actually sabotaging our efforts and increasing our risk of many health problems. High carbohydrate diets (the late 20th-century curse) produce high levels of sugar in the blood, which in turn causes heavy insulin production to move the sugar into the muscle cells or into the liver for later use. If the liver storage cells are full, the insulin will convert the excess blood sugar to a fatty substance called triglyceride, the main constituent in adipose tissue or body fat (Atkins, *Dr. Atkins' New Diet Revolution*, p. 50). When we consume an excess of carbohydrates, we force insulin to store that excess as fat. The reason so many of us are fat is because our diets are too high in carbohydrates, especially refined carbohydrates.

A 12-week study conducted by the Harvard School of Public Health and presented at a meeting of the American Association for the Study of Obesity charted the effects of three diets on three different groups. Group one ate a 1500-calorie low-carb diet and had an average weight loss of 23 pounds. Group two also ate a 1500-calorie diet but it was low fat. Their average weight loss was 17 pounds. The third group was given a low-carb diet with an extra 300 calories. The average weight loss in this 1800-calorie group was 20 pounds. The low-carb group lost more weight while eating more calories than the low fat group.

Some of the meal plans and recipes included in this book recommend increasing the amount of fat you currently consume. For many of you this will be a frightening prospect because for the past three decades you have been told that fat is bad. But Dr. Walter Willett, in his book *Eat, Drink, and Be Healthy*, corrects this by stating, "We have lost sight of the critical fact that not all fats are the same. Or, to put it more bluntly, not all fats are bad. In spite of the scorn heaped upon dietary fat and the anti-fat recommendations from the country's leading health organizations, the truth is that some fats are good for you, and it is important to include these fats in your diet. In fact, eating more good fats and staying away from bad ones is second only to weight control on the list of healthy nutritional strategies" (p. 56). Dr. Willett is a preeminent scientist from the Harvard School of Public Health whose work has made an invaluable contribution to our understanding of nutritional science.

Kinds of Fat

There are four main categories of fat: saturated, monounsaturated, polyunsaturated, and trans fatty acids. Good fats are monounsaturated or polyunsaturated and are often in the liquid forms of olive oil, canola oil, cottonseed oil, and peanut oil. They are also found in cashews, almonds, peanuts, peanut butter, avocados, corn, soybean, safflower, flax seed, and fish. Some good polyunsaturated fats are known medically as "essential fats" because the only way the body can get them is from your diet. These include Omega3 fatty acids found mostly in fish and flaxseed oil and Omega6 fatty acids found in corn, soy, canola, safflower, and sunflower oils. They are essential for building cell membranes and making nerve sheaths, hormones, and chemicals that control blood clotting and muscle contraction (Willett, p. 62).

The bad fats are saturated fats and trans fatty acids. Saturated fats are found in high quantities in whole milk, butter, cheese, ice cream, fatty red meat, chocolate, coconuts, coconut milk, and coconut oil. The trans fatty acids are found in most margarines, vegetable shortening, partially hydrogenated vegetable oil, deep-fried foods, many fast foods, and most commercial baked goods. They are also found in products like peanut butter where they are used to improve smoothness and shelf life. Read the labels carefully to avoid these fats. Anything that is identified as hydrogenated or partially hydrogenated is a trans fatty acid.

An article in *Postgraduate Medicine* in August 2002 stated, "Trans fatty acids increase LDL *(bad)* cholesterol levels to the same extent as saturated fat; the difference is that trans fatty acid intake also decreases HDL *(good)* cholesterol levels, whereas saturated fat typically raises them. The overall result is that the adverse effect of trans fatty acids on the ratio of LDLC to HDLC is double the effect of saturated fat. . . . It appears that long-term Coronary Artery Disease risk is more than doubled in persons who consume a diet high in trans fatty acids."

A report from the *American Journal of Medicine* in December 2002 stated that when carbohydrates are used to replace saturated fats in a low fat diet, both the LDL and HDL components of cholesterol are reduced in similar amounts. This means the ratio between the two types of cholesterol is not improved. It is necessary to improve the ratio if we want to reduce cardiovascular risk.

Consumption of good fats reduces your chance of heart disease and achieves the following benefits:

- lower levels of low density lipoprotein (ldl), a.k.a. bad cholesterol
- higher levels of high density lipoprotein (hdl), a.k.a. good cholesterol
- avoidance of triglycerides that are the result of high carbohydrate intake
- reduced development of erratic heartbeats, the main cause of cardiac death
- reduced likelihood of blood clots in arteries.

These benefits, and those achieved by decreasing your overall carbohydrate intake and choosing slow carbs, are in addition to the health gains made by losing weight. As Dr. Willett says, "next to whether you smoke, the number that stares up at you from the bathroom scale is the most important measure of your future health" (p. 35).

The Healthy Eating Pyramid

Official guides to healthy eating like Canada's Food Guide or the U.S. Department of Agriculture (USDA) Food Guide Pyramid are outdated compared to Dr. Willett's Healthy Eating Pyramid. These older guides consider all fats to be bad and thus recommend they be eaten only sparingly. The Healthy Eating Pyramid (HEP) puts good fats at the base of the pyramid to be consumed at virtually every meal. Previous guides placed carbohydrates such as bread, cereal, rice, and pasta at the base of the pyramid to constitute 6 to 11 servings per day. The HEP places those foods at the top of the pyramid and suggests they be eaten infrequently and in small quantity. Furthermore, Dr. Willett's pyramid puts potatoes and sweets in the same category as bread, cereal, rice, and pasta. Simply put, Dr. Willett has turned the pyramid upside down.

In the January 2003 issue of *Scientific American* he writes,

> How did the USDA pyramid go so wrong? In part nutritionists fell victim to a desire to simplify their dietary recommendations. Researchers had known for decades that saturated fat found in abundance in red meat and dairy products raises cholesterol levels in the blood. High cholesterol levels, in turn, are associated with a high risk

of coronary artery disease (heart attacks and other ailments caused by the blockage of arteries to the heart). In the 1960s, controlled feeding studies, in which the participants eat carefully prescribed diets for several weeks, substantiated that saturated fat increases cholesterol levels. But the studies also showed that polyunsaturated fat found in vegetable oils and fish reduces cholesterol. Thus, dietary advice during the 1960s and 1970s emphasized the replacement of saturated fat with polyunsaturated fat, not total fat reduction. (The subsequent doubling of polyunsaturated fat consumption among Americans probably contributed greatly to the halving of coronary heart disease rates in the U.S. during the 1970s and 1980s.)

Unfortunately, many nutritionists decided it would be too difficult to educate the public about these subtleties. Instead they put out a clear, simple message: 'Fat is bad.' Because saturated fat represents about 40 percent of all fat consumed in the U.S., the rationale of the USDA was that advocating a low fat diet would naturally reduce the intake of saturated fat. This recommendation was soon reinforced by the food industry, which began selling cookies, chips, and other products that were low in fat but often high in sweeteners such as high fructose corn syrup.

When the food pyramid was being developed, the typical American got about 40 percent of his or her calories from fat, about 15 percent from protein, and 45 percent from carbohydrates. Nutritionists did not want to suggest eating more protein, because many sources of protein (red meat, for example) are also heavy in saturated fat. So the 'Fat is bad' mantra led to the corollary 'Carbs are good.' Dietary guidelines from the American Heart Association and other groups recommended that people get at least half of their calories from carbohydrates and no more than 30 percent from fat. This 30 percent limit has become so entrenched among nutritionists that even the sophisticated observer could be forgiven for thinking that many studies must show that individuals with that level of fat intake enjoyed better health than those with higher levels. But no study has demonstrated long-term health benefits that can be directly attributed to a low fat diet. The 30 percent limit on fat was essentially drawn from thin air.

Slow Carb Meets the Mediterranean Diet

Much has been written in medical and nutritional journals about the health benefits of the traditional Mediterranean diet. *The New England Journal of Medicine* reported in its June 26, 2003, issue that a study of 22,043 adults over approximately four years put this to the test. "The traditional Mediterranean diet is characterized by a high intake of vegetables, legumes, fruits and nuts, and cereals (that in the past were largely unrefined), and a high intake of olive oil but a low intake of saturated lipids, a moderately high intake of fish (depending on the proximity of the sea), a low-to-moderate intake of dairy products (and then mostly in the form of cheese or yogurt), a low intake of meat and poultry, and a regular but moderate intake of ethanol, primarily in the form of wine and generally during meals."

Dr. Hu reported in the same issue of *The New England Journal of Medicine* that "evidence suggests that higher dietary Glycemic Load (GL) has adverse effects on blood lipids and is associated with an increased risk of coronary heart disease but that whole grains are beneficial; thus, the effects of cereal intake may depend on the degree of processing. Higher levels of olive oil are considered the hallmark of the traditional Mediterranean diet. For centuries, olive oil has been treasured for its healing and nutritional properties and may have a role in prevention of coronary disease and several types of cancer because of its high levels of monounsaturated fatty acids and polyphenolic compounds. It is worth noting that traditional diets from the Mediterranean and Asian countries share most dietary characteristics, such as a relatively high intake of fruits, vegetables, nuts, legumes, and minimally processed grains, despite use of different sources of plant oils."

Still, most of us have difficulty accepting that eating some fats or fatty food can be good for us. This is why, until recently, so many have been critical of the Atkins diet. How could we possibly eat that way and not increase our cholesterol level? Dr. Eric Westman and his colleagues at Duke University published, in the

American Journal of Medicine in July 2002, the first scientific study of the popular low-carbohydrate Atkins diet in two decades. Study participants were put on a very low-carbohydrate diet of 25 grams per day for six months. They could eat an unlimited amount of meat and eggs, as well as two cups of salad, and one cup of low-carbohydrate vegetables, such as broccoli and cauliflower, a day. Researchers found that 80 percent of the 50 enrolled patients adhered to the diet program for the duration of the study and lost an average of 10 percent of their body weight. The average amount of weight lost per person was approximately 20 pounds. The study further showed that patients' cholesterol levels improved by the end of six months: "We were somewhat surprised to find that the patients' blood lipid profiles improved, even though there was much more fat in the diet. We had thought the fat in the diet would increase the cholesterol." Although exercise was recommended, it was not a requirement for the study. Half of the subjects didn't exercise at all and still lost weight. The results of the study created a media frenzy and accelerated the diet revolution already underway.

A scientific paper published in the *American Journal of Clinical Nutrition* in January 2002 by authors from the Universities of California, Berkeley, and San Francisco concluded that the low fat, high carbohydrate diet was less than ideal, as it could induce liver fat production (triglycerides) and insulin resistance. This was especially true when most of the carbohydrate intake consisted of sugar. A letter to the editor in the April 1, 2003, edition of the *Canadian Medical Association Journal* cited previous research that showed a low fat diet actually increased the levels of triglycerides, blood fats that are associated with an increased risk of heart disease and are a central component to the collection of body fat. "An alternative approach is to radically reduce consumption of all grains and simple sugars. In contrast to the pharmacological options that are traditionally applied, it is simple and inexpensive to substitute green leafy vegetables, which have a low Glycemic Index (GI), for grains and sugars, and there are no toxic effects."

Slow Carb for Life takes this, literally, to heart. Instead of recommending a radical reduction in the consumption of all grains, we recommend elimination of refined grains and a moderate intake of whole grains. We also recommend increasing consumption of good fats and reducing consumption of bad fats.

Dr. Rick: Calgary, Alberta

February 7, 2003

Today, my cardiologist, Jim Stone, has given me a target BMI (Body Mass Index) of 27 so I need to lose about 25–30 pounds. Stone is a prevention-focused cardiologist who treats patients before signs of the disease occur. That's why I had the CT (special x-rays) of my coronary arteries taken — and found they were consistent with someone 65! [Dr. Rick was 47 at that time.] Even though I don't smoke and don't have diabetes, and have controlled my blood pressure, I have a very strong family history and my endothelium is not strong. The target LDL will be below 2.0. The target post MI (heart attack) if you have high LDL is 2.6 (most are 3.4 or higher). He was very clear in pointing out that increased weight would still be a risk even with normal BP and LDL. Thus my journey begins.

March 21, 2003

I got my lipid profile done after six weeks eating low-carb and prior to starting the statin [medical prescription]. I was very interested to see what it was going to be after eating 10 eggs per week, doubling my cheese intake, and quadrupling my nut intake. I was exercising almost daily versus two or three times per week in the winter.

May 15, 2003

Here are my test results 14 weeks after starting to eat low-carb and eight weeks after being on mild medication. These test results are posted in bold for ease of comparison.

The new Canadian guidelines will target the ratio in lipid treatment. It will vary from less than seven for people with no risk factors to less than three for those with extremely high risk. For me, being in the TC/HDL ratio range of 3.5 to 4 with a LDL of 2.0 or 2.2 is the goal. Therefore, after six weeks I added the low dose statin medication. I expected that with this eating lifestyle and only a modest response to the lowest dose of medication a target TC of close to 3.0 and ratio of 3.5 should be easily obtained.

Bottom line: I was truly amazed at the results after six weeks. Sixteen pounds lost and a dramatic improvement in lipid profile despite eating what were once considered the bad foods. I was astonished by the results after 14 weeks. I have exceeded my expectations by far. I am now converted. I also need to buy new belts.

	Normal Range	In the past	After 6 weeks	**After 14 weeks**
Total Cholesterol	3.8 to 5.2	4.8 to 5.1	4.0	**2.16**
Triglycerides	Less than 2.3	2.0 to 2.9	1.1	**0.75**
HDL	More than 0.9	0.6 to 0.7	0.87	**0.89**
LDL	Less than 3.4	3.6 to 4.9	2.66	**0.93**
TC/HDL ratio	Less than 4	6 to 7	4.6	**2.5**

Authors' Note: Dr. Rick went on to lose a total of 40 pounds and he is well established in his maintenance program with risk factors remaining at a very healthy level. His cravings for carbs are gone. He has recommended our books to over 20 of his obese patients, who are frequent visitors to our Web site. In addition to weight loss in excess of five percent of body weight, every one of them has had an improved lipid profile and reduced blood sugar level.

HEALTHY
WEIGHT LOSS

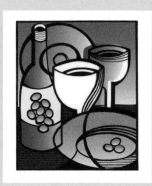

Healthy Weight Loss

The decision to take control of your weight, and your health, is the first and most important step in changing the rest of your life. Once you have made this commitment, there are many things you can do to prepare yourself and make the transition easier. If you reduce your overall carbohydrates, choose slow carbs rather than fast ones, decrease your intake of bad fats, and increase your consumption of good fats, you will lose weight or maintain your ideal weight more easily. You must be prepared to change your eating habits and food choices if you want to change your weight, your health status, and how you feel. You cannot continue with your former eating habits and achieve the desired results. We provide you with a number of simple tools and guidelines to make these changes easier.

Food Diary

Firstly, it is important you know your current level of carbohydrate consumption. We recommend that for the next week, perhaps while you are reading this book, you keep a Food Diary to document your current eating pattern. Make use of the Carb Counter at the end of this book to determine the carb content of the foods you eat. Charting your current carbohydrate consumption for a full week will provide you with a reference to help determine how many grams of carbohydrate you can consume to lose weight. Your target carb level will vary depending on your individual metabolism, current weight, and activity level. Keeping a Food Diary may be the single most important thing you can do to track your food choices.

Keeping track of your food is not as difficult or as time-consuming as it might sound. We have provided a simple format for you to use in the initial weeks of your slow-carb plan. Recording your food will require discipline to look up the carb content of the foods you consume until you have memorized this information. We recommend that you calculate the total net grams of carb intake each evening so that you see at a glance whether you have stayed within your target range. Recognize bad choices and then reaffirm your commitment to stay within your target the next day. Are you eating the wrong kind of snack foods? Are you indulging too much in the evening? This knowledge can help you fine-tune your plan. Your level of carbohydrate consumption will determine the speed of your weight loss and your Food Diary will make this very clear.

We have provided a Food Diary to record the first week of slow-carb eating here, and an electronic version of the Food Diary is also available on our Web site at www.slowcarbforlife.com. You can design your own Food Diary if you choose. It should include the following basic elements: the date; all the food eaten, separated into meals and snacks; the net grams of carbohydrate for each food, plus daily total; any exercise or activity; comments. The weekly summary should include number of carbs for each day; average daily exercise; weekly average of carbs per day; weekly weigh-in information; comments. Keep your Food Diary in the kitchen to record your intake as the day goes along. It is easy to remember, even when you are not eating at home, once you are in the habit.

Monday Food Diary	Carbs	Tuesday Food Diary	Carbs
Breakfast		Breakfast	
Lunch		Lunch	
Dinner		Dinner	
Snacks		Snacks	
Total Carbs		Total Carbs	
Exercise Notes		Exercise Notes	

Wednesday Food Diary	Carbs	Thursday Food Diary	Carbs
Breakfast		Breakfast	
Lunch		Lunch	
Dinner		Dinner	
Snacks		Snacks	
Total Carbs		Total Carbs	
Exercise Notes		Exercise Notes	

Friday Food Diary	Carbs	Saturday Food Diary	Carbs
Breakfast		Breakfast	
Lunch		Lunch	
Dinner		Dinner	
Snacks		Snacks	
Total Carbs		Total Carbs	
Exercise Notes		Exercise Notes	

Sunday Food Diary	Carbs	TOTALS	Carbs	Exercise
Breakfast		Monday		
		Tuesday		
Lunch		Wednesday		
		Thursday		
Dinner		Friday		
		Saturday		
Snacks		Sunday		
		Weekly Total =		
Total Carbs		Divide by 7 for average carbs per day		
Exercise Notes		Weight this week =		
		Notes		

Weigh-ins

We recommend that you weigh and record your weight on a weekly basis. To get the most accurate record you should pick the same day of the week for your weigh-in and weigh yourself first thing in the morning, before putting on any clothes or eating breakfast.

We do not recommend that you weigh yourself on a daily basis. Weighing yourself too frequently places too much emphasis on the weight loss aspect of your slow-carb lifestyle. You may experience daily fluctuations in weight caused by fluid loss or retention or hormonal changes rather than real weight gain or loss. In addition to weight loss, you will likely also experience positive changes in how you feel and how your clothes fit.

Identifying Your Goals

Now that you know how many carbs you regularly consume per day and what you currently weigh, it is time to identify your goals, both in terms of ideal weight and health benefits. As with most endeavors, it is easier to track your progress if you clearly identify your target and record milestones. Your goal may be as simple as losing 20 pounds. Perhaps you are still unsure about a slow-carb approach and think it better to set a short-term goal of eating slow-carb for two weeks to determine if it is an approach to weight loss you can maintain. Take into account your energy level during this period, your ability to focus during the day, any impact on your exercise plan, your feelings of hunger or satisfaction after a meal, and of course any weight change. The health benefits and initial weight loss should become obvious within two weeks, if you are faithful to the slow-carb approach.

There are many reasons for wanting to lose weight: perhaps there is a family wedding to attend for which you want to improve your appearance, perhaps your doctor has cautioned you to lose weight for medical reasons, or you know from your family history that you are at risk for adult onset diabetes, perhaps you want to improve your energy level. . . . Whatever your reasons, you will find it easier to adhere to your plan if you have taken the time to articulate and record your goals. When you feel you might be lacking resolve, go back to your goals and remind yourself why you decided to start a slow-carb plan. When friends or family are less supportive than you would like, support yourself by referring to your goals and noting your success in working toward them.

Setting Your Daily Carb Intake Level

Many of the more widely known low-carb diets require users to adopt an extremely low level of carbohydrate intake (as low as 20 grams or less per day) during the initial period of two or three weeks. The theory is that a drastic change in diet will force the body into ketosis and shift the metabolism into high gear, which will result in immediate weight loss. We do not believe that it is necessary to restrict your carb intake to less than 20 grams of carb a day, even during weight loss; we recommend between 30 and 50 grams a day. This provides you with flexibility and variety in choosing your foods on a daily basis and will seem less punitive. Slow-carb living is not a diet; it is a way of life.

How do you determine your ideal carbohydrate intake for weight loss? This will depend on how many pounds you want to lose, your own metabolism (women generally have slower metabolisms than men, so men can usually afford to eat a higher intake of carbs and still lose weight), your activity level, how strict you are willing to be with your carb intake, and what time frame you think is reasonable to achieve the desired weight loss. Think about how long it took you to get to where you are today. It didn't happen overnight, or even in a month or two. Be kind to yourself. Be realistic. If you have a large amount of weight to lose, perhaps you can set interim weight goals.

If you restrict your intake of carbs to just 30 grams a day for the first three months of the weight loss program, you'll lose an average of 10 pounds each month, or 2.5 pounds a week. This is rapid weight loss. If you then increase your carb intake to about 45 grams per day, you'll continue losing about a pound a week.

A slow-carbohydrate lifestyle means limiting your carbohydrate intake to foods that slowly turn to blood sugar; it does not mean eliminating carbohydrates from your diet. This would be virtually impossible to do as all foods except proteins and fats contain carbohydrates. Furthermore, a diet without carbohydrates would not be healthy. Vegetables, fruits, grains, nuts, and seeds all contain carbohydrates. On a slow-carb weight loss plan you dramatically reduce the carbohydrates you eat and force the body to burn fat for energy. The real trick is to eat less than you need for your daily routine in order to start burning stored fat. The slow-carb plan that we recommend is not protein-loaded like some of the other low-carb diets. Protein loading may cause calcium to leach from the bones and this is not healthy for anyone, particularly women. Protein loading may also be dangerous for anyone who has kidney disease.

As discussed, the other half of the healthy eating equation is to minimize consumption of bad fats. Get into the habit of choosing fish, pork, or poultry instead of fatty red meats, as none of these foods have significant quantities of saturated fats. Many of the fast foods North Americans consume, especially those that are deep-fried, are cooked in trans fatty acids. French fries, for example, are high in carbohydrate content (35 grams in every 4 ounces of potato), have a high Glycemic Index (GI) of 90 so the Glycemic Load (GL) is 32, and are deep-fried in oil containing trans fatty acids. French fries do not belong in a healthy diet.

We feel that we have developed a plan that is simple in its approach, based on hard science; it is balanced, flexible, and easy to implement. The slow-carb weight loss plan requires that you give up bread, most cereals, potatoes, rice, pasta, and sugar during weight loss. Some of these foods can be gradually reintroduced on a limited basis during maintenance. Fruit is allowed in small portions during weight loss and increasing portions during maintenance. There is no weighing, measuring, calculating points, or counting calories, but you will need to learn to count your carbohydrates.

Simply try the level of carb intake that you think you can handle most easily for a week and track your progress. If you feel you are losing weight too quickly or that you don't have sufficient flexibility, then increase it. If you would like to lose faster, or feel that you don't need the extra flexibility, then you may want to decrease your carb intake. We do not recommend that you take your carb intake below 30 net grams a day.

We would caution you not to lose weight too quickly. If you put on the extra pounds over a period of years, it doesn't make sense to try to take it all off within a couple of weeks. You will probably see a fairly dramatic weight loss, anywhere from five to 10 pounds, in the first week of our slow-carb approach. Much of this will be fluid that your body loses when your system initially switches to burning fat for energy rather than sugar. Once the system adjusts to this switch in metabolism, the weight loss will slow to anywhere from one to two and a half pounds per week. This slower rate will be healthier for you and easier for your body to accommodate. At two and a half pounds a week, you will lose 10 pounds a month! It doesn't take very many months on this plan before you will have lost a significant amount of weight.

When you have reached your ideal weight you will likely require 50 to 100 grams of carb per day to maintain that weight, though this depends on your rate of metabolism and activity level. It is important to remember there are no absolutes — you choose which carbohydrates to eat. Once you have lost the weight you'd like, if you occasionally give in to a burning desire for pizza, you need only modify your intake for the next day or two to stay within your daily average. You may choose to adjust volume as well as variety. For example, you could eat a large salad, or coleslaw and two cups of vegetables, or some fruit, to make up your daily allotment of carbohydrate rather than a single slice of pizza. Remember, you have control.

Carb-Proofing Your Environment

Before you get started, create a safe slow-carb environment in your home; ensure that the foods you have chosen to consume are readily available. Get in a stash of slow-carb snacks — hard-boiled eggs, cheese, celery, nuts, seeds, sugar-free gum, low-carb protein bars, homemade slow-carb bars, slow-carb muffins, protein shakes, cucumbers, yogurt, sugar-free Jell-O — and remove all the packaged baked goods, cake mixes, candy, chocolate, potato chips, corn chips, popcorn, crackers, cereals, cookies, and pretzels. If they are not readily available, it is much easier to do without than to make a special trip in order to get them. If you keep snacks in your desk drawer, make sure that they are of the slow-carb variety. Make your choices easy by eliminating the tempting foods that you no longer want to consume (give it to the food bank or have a party and let all your friends eat it for you!). It is equally important that the people you live with and care about are supportive of your efforts and understand how important these changes are for you.

If you have a family who want access to higher carb foods and snacks, re-organize your kitchen so all the high carb food is kept in one cupboard and then avoid going into it. Although it is easier to prepare and consume slow-carb meals if you don't have to prepare high carb foods for your family, it can be done with some determination and willpower. If you can do this for even a short period of time, you will be so pleased with the results that you will find it easier to continue to exercise good judgment and control your carbohydrate intake. Perhaps you can ask your family to adopt a slow-carb approach in support of your efforts. If there are members of the family who do not want to lose weight, increase their portions of fruits, higher carb vegetables, and certain whole grain products so that they maintain their weight.

Buying (S)low-Carb

If you are the person responsible for food planning, shopping, and preparation and have spent years searching for low fat products, you now must switch your thinking to slow-carb. If you are buying salad dressing, for example, you will want to avoid the low fat variety that adds sugar to increase flavor, making it much higher in carbs than the regular variety.

Both Dr. Atkins and Dr. Barry Sears *(The Zone)* are convinced that reduction in carbs results in more efficient metabolizing of fat. If we eat low-carb, we can actually lose weight while consuming a higher number of calories than we did while eating high-carb. But why not eat a healthy balance of proteins, good fats, and slow carbohydrates that will inevitably reduce the number of daily calories you consume? Do you need to count your calories? Absolutely not. Remember, this is designed to be easy. Simply control your carbs and keep track of them.

For readers who are completely new to the idea of a low-carb kitchen and the ingredients necessary to prepare slow-carb meals, we have developed a list of the basics. You may not need these ingredients all at once or every week, but this is a good place to start.

Slow-Carb Grocery List

eggs

light cream

heavy cream

plain yogurt

cottage cheese

cheddar cheese

butter

balsamic vinegar

olive oil

lettuce or bag of mixed greens

cucumbers

celery

cauliflower

green beans

asparagus

zucchini

carrots

green cabbage

red cabbage

green onion

onion

mushrooms

green pepper

real mayonnaise

lemons

lemon juice

limes

fresh strawberries

kiwi fruit

canned tuna

bacon

boneless skinless chicken breasts

lean ground beef

fresh fish

almonds

sugar-free Jell-O, many flavors

soda water

herb tea

coffee or decaf coffee

Splenda

Here are some ingredients found in our slow-carb muffins and other baked goods that you may find in your health food or specialty store:

Xanthan gum

low-carb protein powder

whey protein powder

soy protein powder

flax seed meal

oat flour

soy flour

Building a Support Team

If you have to deal with friends or family who are skeptical or even negative about your new approach to eating, explain that while you appreciate their concern, you feel you have done the appropriate research and this approach is a healthy alternative for you. Tell them that they don't need to understand it or even try it, but that you would like them to support you in your efforts. You may decide that educating them requires a time commitment you don't want to make, but if you do want to help them understand, this book and those listed in the annotated bibliography are a good place to start.

If you feel your efforts are being sabotaged by those who drop by with warm cinnamon buns during coffee break or a friend who entreats you to "take one little bite" of something you know is not good for you, learn to refuse with good humour, a joke, or a smile. Unfortunately, people may conclude that your behavior is an indirect comment on theirs and become defensive. One way to defuse this situation is to make it a health issue; for example, state that you have a "sensitivity" to wheat and you feel you are healthier when you don't eat baked goods.

Many of us have our own food triggers, an event, an activity, an emotion, or a food or food type that makes us want to eat (or binge) when we are not hungry. Watching television is a food trigger for some, so it is best to limit any snacks during TV time and do some other activity that uses your hands at the same time. Pay attention to your eating habits and take precautions to avoid any foods or situations that might lead you to overindulge.

Once you have made the decision to follow a slow-carb approach to eating, and you explain the why and how of your decision to your family and close friends, you may want to find others attempting the same thing. Check out our Web site, www.slowcarbforlife.com, and other Web sites listed in the support network section that provide a forum for discussion and information about research and new products.

Exercising

Everyone, whether they wish to lose weight or not, should exercise regularly. Physical activity can and should help you to lose weight by burning calories; increasing your metabolic rate; increasing your energy; adding muscle, which burns more calories; reducing the output of insulin; protecting you from heart disease, high blood pressure, high cholesterol, some cancers (colon and breast), adult onset diabetes, arthritis, osteoporosis; relieving symptoms of depression and anxiety; and it can be FUN!

Exercise burns calories otherwise stored as fat and builds muscle. Even while you sleep your muscles continue to use energy (calories). The more muscle mass you have, the more calories are burned. Brisk walking is one of the best exercises and requires only commitment and a good pair of walking shoes to be effective. Dr. Willett reported (p. 51) that in the Nurses' Health Study, women who walked an average of three hours per week at a brisk pace were 35 percent less likely to have a heart attack over an eight-year period than women who walked infrequently. A 30-minute daily walk will go a long way to helping you take off, and keep off, those extra pounds. Consider martial arts, pilates, yoga, volleyball, basketball, hockey — the options are endless.

If you are not accustomed to regular physical activity, the mere thought of it may be daunting. Rick Gallop in his book *The GI Diet* (p. 105–107) lists three common excuses people use to avoid getting started. The first is the excuse that exercising causes pain and discomfort. This is likely a matter of having done too much too soon. If you are going to start walking, don't try doing three miles the first day. Go for a block or two and work up from there — slowly. The second excuse is that exercise is boring. Get creative, listen to music, plan your activity in the company of a friend, ride your stationary bicycle in front of the TV. The third excuse is lack of time. Gallop reminds us that every week has 336 30-minute blocks; if you commit to using two percent of those for exercise you have one block every day. Dr. Anne McTiernan of the Fred Hutchinson Cancer Research Center in Seattle says women in their 30s who are physically active will reduce their risk of breast cancer. Her study found that even a brisk half-hour walk three times a week is enough to lower a woman's cancer risk by about 20 percent.

Guidelines for Slow-Carb Living

The following basic common sense principles about food and food choices apply equally for weight loss and weight maintenance. For readers who have tried other diets and weight loss plans, some of the ideas presented will be familiar.

Do not skip breakfast. Your body has been without nourishment for many hours by the time you get up. You need protein to maintain a blood sugar level that allows you to feel energetic and alert.

Eat frequently and in small portions. We recommend three good meals and two to three snacks each day. Do not skip any meals if you want to experience high energy levels all day. Include protein at every meal and snack (eggs, cheese, meat, chicken, fish, nuts, or seeds).

Avoid high GI carb food. This includes all baked goods (pies, cakes, cookies, doughnuts), white breads, bagels, muffins, scones; candy; most cereal; corn, beets, peas, beans, and lentils; fruit juices; bananas, apples, oranges; pasta; potatoes, sweet potatoes; rice; and sugar.

Keep slow-carb foods in the fridge. These should be readily available, whether for snacks or as part of a meal. These include cheese, cottage cheese (dry curd, creamed or 4 percent fat), yogurt (whole); dairy products including butter, light cream, whole milk, and heavy cream (in moderate amounts during weight loss); eggs and egg substitutes; fish, shellfish; extra virgin olive oil, canola oil, peanut oil; lemons, limes; pork, bacon, lamb, veal, and lean cuts of red meat; nuts and seeds; chicken, turkey, or other fowl; tofu and other soy products; lettuce, celery, cucumber, all sprouts, garlic, Swiss chard, okra, spinach, mushrooms, green cabbage, red cabbage, cauliflower, asparagus, avocado, broccoli, green beans, yellow beans, zucchini, eggplant, summer and spaghetti squash.

Eat a daily serving of fruit. Be careful in your choices and your portions, especially during weight loss. Try strawberries, raspberries, blackberries, kiwi fruit, grapefruit, or peaches.

Drink at least eight glasses of water every day. As with any weight loss plan, it is important to keep your body hydrated and to facilitate the flushing of waste products. If you do not like the taste of tap water, try filtered water, bottled water, or soda water. Herb teas are naturally decaffeinated and are better than regular teas that may contribute to the formation of kidney stones when consumed in large quantities.

Avoid soft drinks. A single can of Coke has approximately 39 grams of carbohydrate in it — more than we recommend at the lower level of carb intake for your entire day during weight loss. Diet drinks do not have any carbohydrates, but most of them still contain aspartame as the sweetening agent (see next page). Some diet soft drink manufacturers have switched to Splenda as the sweetening agent, but check the label.

Drink alcohol in moderation. There is growing evidence that one or two drinks per day contribute to heart health, but no alcohol is better than too much. A glass of wine has approximately four grams of carb, and spirits mixed with water have zero carbs. If you consume mixed drinks, it is the mix that is high in carbohydrates. Beer has 13 grams of carb per 12 ounce bottle, though there are some new "low-carb" beers that have reduced their carb content to about three grams.

Avoid caffeine. Caffeine stimulates the pancreas to produce insulin, which is counterproductive and can stimulate hunger, so you may wish to switch to decaffeinated coffee in the morning or later in the day. If you use light cream use it sparingly, and if you prefer a sweetener we recommend Splenda.

Watch the carb count of sauces and dressings. Carbohydrates can add up quickly when you add salad dressing. Be sure to purchase regular or low-carb salad dressings rather than the low fat variety. You can garnish salads with hard-boiled eggs, cheese, nuts, and sunflower seeds to add taste and protein without adding dramatically to the carb count. Garlic, most herbs, mustard, real mayonnaise, olives, salt and pepper, or vinegar are also good choices. Do not use ketchup, jams, mint jelly, or applesauce, all of which contain sugar and therefore are high in carbs. Sugar-free and no sugar added garnishes and sauces are available in your grocery store.

Sugar Substitutes

There are a number of sugar substitutes on the market. The one we use and recommend is sucralose, marketed under the name of Splenda. It is our opinion that none of the other options offer any advantage over Splenda and most have definite disadvantages. We present our reasons in the discussion that follows.

Sucralose (Splenda). Splenda is made from sugar. Its scientific name is sucralose, and it can best be described as a sugar derivative. The chemical process that converts sugar to sucralose changes the sugar molecule so that it cannot be digested by the body. Because it is not digested it doesn't stimulate the release of insulin. Splenda doesn't change either its consistency or its flavor when heated, which makes it suitable for baking and cooking. Splenda is the only sugar substitute that has been recommended by *Health* magazine. There is no aspartame or other chemicals or additives in Splenda.

Splenda is available in three or four forms, depending on your location. The liquid form is not currently available in North America, although lobbyists are trying to convince the company to make it available. Small individual packets, boxed granular Splenda, and individual tablets for hot drinks are available. Use packets for convenience when cooking and baking or the loose granular sugar when the recipe calls for bulk. Splenda in packets is concentrated and is equivalent to two teaspoons of sugar. Granulated Splenda is not concentrated and may be used in quantities equal to sugar when substituting in a favorite recipe.

Aspartame (Equal, Nutrasweet). Until Splenda came along, aspartame was the most widely used artificial sweetener. It replaced saccharin largely because it did not stimulate the release of insulin. However, it does not remain stable when heated, so it is difficult to use in cooking. It can also cause headaches, indigestion, sleep disturbances, and dizziness. Scientific evidence and anecdotal reports also suggest it can be a risk to the brain and nervous system as can monosodium glutamate (MSG). However, it is still widely used as an artificial sweetener, especially in soft drinks.

Saccharin (Sweet 'N Low). This is the oldest of the artificial sweeteners (discovered in 1879) and though it was mostly replaced by aspartame, it probably is still a better option. It has few side effects and remains stable when heated so it can be used in cooking. A major disadvantage is that it stimulates the pancreas to release insulin. Laboratory studies using high doses in rats did produce bladder cancer but this has never happened in humans. In our opinion there is minimal health risk if you occasionally want to use Sweet 'N Low as your sweetener.

Cyclamate (Sugar Twin, Sucaryl). Cyclamate remains stable in heat so it is useful for cooking. This product is available in Canada but remains banned in the United States because of concerns about bladder cancer in rats. This has never been shown in humans despite 30 years of study. The occasional use of this sweetener poses no serious health risk.

Stevia. This is a natural sweetener sold primarily in health food stores. It remains stable in liquids and heat so can be used to sweeten drinks or for cooking and baking. It does have a slight licorice flavor and is extremely sweet, which makes it difficult to determine the proper amount to use in a recipe. This natural sweetener can stimulate the release of insulin so should be used sparingly.

Sugar Alcohols (maltitol, sorbitol, xylitol). These products are not absorbed in the intestine so they do not stimulate the release of insulin, but they can cause a laxative effect, so use with caution. New low-carb products, "diabetic" candies, gums, and sugar-free chocolate products also use them as sweeteners. The carb content of sugar-free chocolates can vary from 3 or 4 grams to 15 to 17 grams per chocolate so check the packaging.

Meal Plans for Weight Loss

Knowing how to plan meals that will be tasty and nutritious as well as slow-carb is a challenge for most people beginning the slow-carb plan. Having a variety of easy-to-prepare recipes will take some of the guesswork out of the decision making for you. The following seven daily menus for slow-carb weight loss provide you with a sample that is varied and includes three meals and two snacks per day. Try to keep snacks to three or four grams of carb and don't forget to include them in your Food Diary. We have tried to develop lunch menus that can be taken to work or eaten at home and that use the leftover protein from the evening meal the preceding day. We have included a number of kinds of muffins (for those who miss their breads!) and suggest you bake several types in advance and freeze them.

Some of the recipes used in the Meal Plans are contained in the Recipes section of this book. All of the recipes are contained in *All New Easy Low-Carb Cooking*. It is normal to feel hungry before we eat. It is also normal to feel you are eating less than you used to while following the weight loss plan. If you still feel hungry after a meal, then you are not eating enough. Add green salads and other low-carb vegetables to satisfy you. The hunger should gradually abate as your system adjusts to metabolizing slow-carbohydrate foods. During the weight loss phase we recommend that you try to stick to foods that you have prepared, using these recipes (as opposed to pre-packaged low-carb foods). All of the daily menus have been developed to maintain a carbohydrate content of between 30 and 50 grams of net carb a day. In our calculation of net carb, we have subtracted only the fiber content of foods.

Weight Loss Menu Plan

DAY ONE

		Net Carbohydrates
Breakfast	2 eggs, scrambled	1.2
	2 slices of bacon	0.0
	coffee, light cream	0.5
Snack	Walnut Flax Muffin	2.4
	decaf coffee, light cream	0.5
Lunch	Tuna Salad	1.8
	Fancy Coleslaw	3.5
	1/2 cup raspberries	2.9
	water, herb tea	0.0
Snack	1 oz cheddar cheese	0.0
Dinner	Grilled Herb Chicken	2.1
	Grilled Zucchini	2.1
	1/2 cup steamed broccoli	1.7
	Grapefruit & Spinach Salad	6.7
	1/2 cup sliced strawberries	3.6
Total Net Carbohydrates		29.0

DAY TWO

		Net Carbohydrates
Breakfast	1/2 cup cottage cheese	2.0
	1/2 cup sliced strawberries	3.6
	coffee, light cream	0.5
Snack	Orange Cranberry Muffin	4.9
	decaf coffee, light cream	0.5
Lunch	Oriental Chicken Salad	11.6
	sugar-free Jell-O	0.0
Snack	Walnut Flax Muffin	2.4
Dinner	Poached Salmon with Citrus Sauce	4.2
	1/2 cup steamed cauliflower	0.8
	Green Beans with Mustard	0.9
	Fancy Coleslaw	3.5
	1/2 cup raspberries	2.9
Total Net Carbohydrates		37.8

DAY THREE

		Net Carbohydrates
Breakfast	2 eggs, poached	2.0
	1 slice ham	0.0
	coffee, light cream	0.5
Snack	Ham & Cheese Roll-Up	1.7
	decaf coffee, light cream	0.5
Lunch	Salmon Salad	2.1
	1/2 cup lettuce	1.0
	1/2 cup cucumber slices	1.0
	2 tablespoons Red Wine Vinaigrette	1.2
	1/2 cup strawberries	3.6
Snack	Chocolate Nut Protein Bar	6.4
Dinner	Teriyaki Burger	1.6
	1/2 cup steamed broccoli	1.7
	Grilled Eggplant	4.9
	Easy Coleslaw	2.1
	1/2 cup raspberries	2.9
Total Net Carbohydrates		33.2

DAY FOUR

		Net Carbohydrates
Breakfast	1/2 cup whole plain yogurt	5.0
	1/2 cup sliced strawberries	3.6
	coffee, light cream	0.5
Snack	1 hard boiled egg	1.0
	decaf coffee, light cream	0.5
Lunch	Cold Teriyaki Burger	1.6
	Easy Coleslaw	2.1
	1/2 cup raspberries	2.9
Snack	Oatmeal Flax Muffin	4.1
Dinner	Roast Chicken with Lemon & Rosemary	0.2
	1/2 cup steamed asparagus	1.9
	Creamy Garlic Cauliflower	3.0
	Broccoli Salad	5.7
	sugar-free Jell-O	0.0
Total Net Carbohydrates		32.1

DAY FIVE

		Net Carbohydrates
Breakfast	Mushroom & Spinach Frittata	3.1
	coffee, light cream	0.5
Snack	Chocolate Nut Protein Bar	6.4
	decaf coffee, light cream	0.5
Lunch	Spinach Salad	4.4
	sugar-free Jell-O	0.0
Snack	Oatmeal Flax Muffin	4.1
	diet soft drink	0.0
Dinner	cold roast chicken	0.5
	Red Cabbage Casserole	6.9
	Green Beans with Mustard	0.9
	Broccoli Salad	5.7
	1/2 cup raspberries	2.9
Total Net Carbohydrates		35.9

DAY SIX

		Net Carbohydrates
Breakfast	Easy Cheesy Quiche	4.2
	Oatmeal Pumpkin Muffin	4.6
	coffee, light cream	0.5
Snack	1 celery stick, 1 tbsp. peanut butter	2.5
	decaf coffee, light cream	0.5
Lunch	(cold) Mushroom & Spinach Frittata	3.1
	1/2 Spinach Salad	2.2
	sugar-free Jell-O	0.0
Snack	Citrus Protein Bar	4.5
Dinner	Steamed Halibut with Herbs & Vegetables	4.4
	1/2 cup steamed green beans	2.9
	Savory Coleslaw	2.5
	1/2 cup raspberries	2.9
Total Net Carbohydrates		34.8

DAY SEVEN

		Net Carbohydrates
Breakfast	Easy Cheesy Quiche (reheated)	4.2
	Orange Cranberry Muffin	4.9
	coffee, light cream	0.5
Snack	Citrus Protein Bar	4.5
	decaf coffee, light cream	0.5
Lunch	Waldorf Salad	5.6
	sugar-free Jell-O	0.0
Snack	1 oz. cheddar cheese	0.0
Dinner	Peppered Steak	0.6
	Green Beans with Bacon & Mushrooms	5.1
	Creamy Garlic Cauliflower	3.0
	Savory Coleslaw	2.5
	1/2 cup sliced strawberries	3.6
Total Net Carbohydrates		35.0

Weight Loss Plateau

As with other weight loss and weight management programs, the body will sometimes adapt or adjust over time to the new level of food intake. This can cause your weight loss to stall or plateau. If you are losing one pound a week you are not stalled, although you may be losing more slowly than you prefer. This is a very respectable weight loss and within a few months you will be noticeably thinner. A plateau occurs when you have been losing weight consistently and then level off and maintain your weight for at least three weeks without any further decrease. It may be that your body has adapted to your new eating habits or has gone into starvation mode because it fears it will not be fed again. This may be an easy plateau to fix, by adding more bulk to your daily intake of food, especially in the form of greens and vegetables. This is counterintuitive, but adding food to your meal plan can encourage the body to get back to weight loss.

Refer to your Food Diary to determine what sort of strategy or change is necessary to kick-start the weight loss. The discipline that keeping a Food Diary involves is particularly important at the beginning when you are making major changes in your habits and adjusting to a new way of thinking about food. It is too easy to lose track of your carb intake if you are not writing things down. All the little extras and snacks will add up quickly, or you'll simply forget that you decided to have a piece of Aunt Bertha's birthday cake. When you write this down, you are reminded to have a low-carb day the next day to compensate for your splurge. This will help keep you on track and may avoid the disappointment of small gains. Recording your activity level in your Food Diary will also help to identify any change in activity level that may have contributed to a plateau in weight loss.

There are many foods that can cause a weight loss plateau. One of the likely suspects is the commercial low-carb bar or any of the other new products that advertise "net carbs," so we suggest you eliminate these first. Other foods that can cause a plateau include anything with a high salt content (salted nuts, salted seeds, and pork rinds). If you want to continue to eat nuts you may choose to try the roasted, but unsalted variety, or try natural raw nuts and seeds. Some individuals report that foods with artificial sweeteners cause a plateau or trigger cravings for additional sweets.

If it is not immediately obvious what has caused the plateau, you need to engage in a process of trial and error to see if you can identify the culprit. Are you getting enough exercise? If not, try adding a 30-minute walk on a daily basis. Are you snacking in the evening after dinner? Try some sugar-free Jell-O or sugar-free gum before bed. Reduce your daily carb intake to something just a bit lower to get your metabolism back into high gear. Add some additional vegetables (the slow-carb variety) and salads to add bulk to your meals. Or maybe you just need to be patient. We have known individuals to plateau for as many as six or eight weeks for no apparent reason, and then suddenly start losing again. Keep your consumption of carbs to the level that you have determined works best and eventually you will be rewarded.

A small percentage of people experience some side effects when they start the slow-carb approach to eating. There is no clinical evidence to determine why this happens, but it may be that some of you are more susceptible to withdrawal symptoms when you eliminate foods like wheat, sugar, or caffeine. If you experience headaches, upset stomach, or light-headedness, you might want to slowly eliminate these foods from your diet rather than do it all in one fell swoop. Try drinking a couple of cups of coffee for a few days, then reduce your intake to just one cup a day. It will be easier for you to adapt to this level of restriction, and your body will not react so dramatically.

Some individuals experience slight or moderate constipation when they start a slow-carb meal plan. Eat plenty of leafy green vegetables to increase your fiber intake or try a high-fiber cereal like All Bran Extra Fiber or muffins made with flax seed meal. Sprinkle flax seed meal or flax seeds on yogurt or salads to add fiber. Finally, eat fruit with your morning meal to help with regularity.

If you do experience any of these minor side effects, just be patient and the symptoms should abate in a few days. Once you are established in your slow-carb lifestyle you may occasionally experience headaches following a sugar splurge because the body no longer tolerates the sugar consumption it used to.

Grandma: Qualicum Beach, British Columbia

In September I weighed 230 pounds. I had tried low fat diets and any increase in exercise has always been extremely painful (old injuries, possible fibromyalgia according to my doctor). I was having difficulty keeping up with my young grandchildren, and was wondering if I could work full time for the next five years (until I retired at age 60). So in a last ditch effort, I hired a trainer. She advised a low-carb diet, eating protein at every meal, and drinking lots of water. Also, I started on a low-impact regime at the gym. After six weeks of minimal exercise, my body was still in a lot of pain, although I had started to lose weight. I thought I would try aquafit at the pool. I continued to lose weight, although more slowly. I now weigh 188 pounds. My weight loss pattern was to lose one or two pounds a week, then my weight would stay the same for about two weeks (for no apparent reason) and then start going down again. My weight has stayed the same for the last four weeks, so I was interested in reading about this phenomena in your book, and I will reevaluate what I am doing/not doing. I plan to buy your cookbook as soon as I can.

EFFECTIVE WEIGHT MAINTENANCE

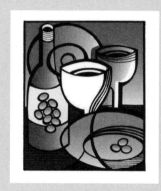

Effective Weight Maintenance

Most of the information in our book focuses on weight loss and weight maintenance because that is what frequently motivates people to make changes in their diet. However, *Slow Carb for Life* is also for those who do not need to lose weight, but do wish to adopt healthy eating habits in order to maintain their weight.

Once you have achieved your ideal weight (weekly weigh-ins) and your daily average carbohydrate intake is consistent, you know exactly how many carbs you can ingest on average without gaining weight. Your Food Diary should be a useful summary document and a reassuring tool when you reach this maintenance phase. Though weight maintenance is now your primary goal, it is still important to weigh yourself weekly to ensure that you are not losing or gaining significant amounts. You may lose an additional two or three pounds if you have a very active week and burn up more energy than usual. Without a regular schedule of weigh-ins, you may not be alerted to this small loss. If this happens, simply increase your carbohydrate intake the following week (often with the addition of extra fruit servings) to regain those few pounds. A small loss, if it happens on an isolated basis, is not a major concern, but if you have successive weeks of high activity levels and the associated losses, you might find yourself below your ideal weight.

The beauty of the slow-carb approach to weight control is that you don't have to dramatically change the eating habits you developed during weight loss. There are no new rules or significant changes to food choices or food preparation beyond increasing your daily intake of slow carbs until you find the level at which you maintain your ideal weight. The transition should be seamless once you find your individual tolerance level. In this way you can continue to eat slow-carb foods with greater flexibility, but without putting on the weight you worked so hard to lose.

Increasing Your Carb Intake

When we talk about increasing your intake of slow carbs we do not mean that you can return to your old habits of eating white bread, potatoes, and pasta. You can occasionally enjoy brown rice, whole-wheat pasta, and whole grain products without unwanted spikes in blood sugar levels and loss of energy or weight gain. You can also increase the number of servings of fruit you enjoy as it provides many vitamins and other nutrients our bodies require to function at an optimum level. Fruit also introduces natural sweetness and makes an ideal snack or dessert. Many of you will want to eat whole grains that are slow carbs and have a low Glycemic Load (GL), but do not eat refined grains or their products (white breads and anything made with refined white flour). You may also want to indulge in some slow-carb desserts at this stage. You will notice that in our menu plans some of them are a little higher in carb content than others, but we have been careful to control your daily carb intake to accommodate this so there is no adverse effect on your weight or your health.

Metabolism and activity level will affect exactly how many grams of carb you can consume for maintenance. To determine your individual tolerance levels, we suggest that you start by increasing your daily carb intake by 10 grams a day. For example, if you have been losing weight at 40 grams a day, you should start your transition to maintenance at 50 grams a day. Maintain an accurate Food Diary and at the end of your first week of transition weigh yourself. Did you continue to lose? Even a weight loss of half a pound indicates that you need to increase your carb intake further. A weight loss of one or two pounds indicates that you are well below the carb intake levels you require so add another 10 grams per day. Your scale will direct you to the target level for the next week. It may take three or four weeks before you reach a carb intake level suitable for consistent weight. In general, we recommend somewhere between 50 and 100 grams of carb a day. Greater flexibility and variety in your foods and room for the occasional indulgence is not, however, licence to return to your old habits. Start your transition slowly, learning how your body reacts to the introduction of these foods. Continue to read food labels and purchase the same types of foods that you ate during weight loss.

Controlling your carbohydrates at your new target level will allow you to eat well without gaining any of the weight you worked so hard to lose. You should not yo-yo when you stop the weight loss period, nor should you have to closely monitor portion control so that you feel you are on a diet. Because you will be eating like this on a regular basis, choose foods that you enjoy so there is no hardship and your motivation level remains high. Note that some foods you were able to eat without any obvious adverse effects prior to eating slow-carb may now produce headaches, weight gain, bloating, fatigue, and digestive upset. The body may react more dramatically to a food or an ingredient if it has not been part of the daily diet for some time. An extreme response may signal that this is a food you should avoid, even in small amounts.

Exercise Routines

During your transition to weight maintenance your Food Diary should reflect your physical activity level. Your metabolism will increase in direct proportion to the activity. Walking, running, yoga, pilates, martial arts, biking, hiking, or any other activity you enjoy will require energy your body will draw from your carb intake or from your stored fat. Remember, to have a healthy lifestyle we require regular exercise.

Introducing New Low-Carb Products

You may now wish to experiment with specialty low-carb products increasingly found on supermarket shelves and in low-carb stores. This approach has become so popular that manufacturers are developing new products to keep up with increased demand. That said, be careful if these products use sugar alcohols (like maltitol) in their preparation. If they do, they may have a laxative effect if ingested in sufficient quantities (varies according to metabolism). Some people may absorb either the glycerine or sugar alcohols used in these products, which can cause weight gain and the return of food cravings. Do not eat these products every day, but one every week or every other week should be fine to start. Monitor your response to low-carb products by maintaining an accurate Food Diary and regular weigh-ins. We think it is preferable to increase your carb intake with fresh foods or home-baked muffins, breads, and desserts.

Meal Plans for Everyday

We have prepared a week-long menu plan suitable for slow-carb maintenance featuring meals that vary between 40 and 60 grams of net carb per day. If you are active or have a high metabolism, you may need more than 60 grams per day. Each day contains three full meals and two snacks. A small snack may be added before bedtime, if necessary, but make sure that it has fewer than five grams of net carb. We have deducted fiber content to arrive at the net carb figure. Drink as much water and herb tea as you like with these menus.

Weight Maintenance Menu Plan

DAY ONE

		Net Carbohydrates
Breakfast	oatmeal, 1/4 cup light cream	13.0
	coffee, light cream	0.5
Snack	Ham & Cheese Roll-Up	1.7
	decaf coffee, light cream	0.5
Lunch	(cold) Lemon Herb Chicken	1.3
	Oriental Coleslaw	4.8
	sugar-free Jell-O	0.0
Snack	1/4 cup almonds	1.0
Dinner	Meat Loaf with Tomato Sauce	3.5
	Creamy Garlic Cauliflower	3.0
	1/2 cup steamed green beans	2.9
	Salmon and Avocado Salad	4.0
	peach	7.1
Total Net Carbohydrates		43.3

DAY TWO

		Net Carbohydrates
Breakfast	All Bran Extra Fiber	
	with 1/4 cup light cream	7.0
	coffee, light cream	0.5
Snack	Chocolate Nut Protein Bar	6.4
	decaf coffee, light cream	0.5
Lunch	Meat Loaf (reheated)	3.5
	Tangy Coleslaw	2.1
	1/2 cup sliced strawberries	3.6
Snack	Slice of Walnut Pumpkin Loaf	4.2
Dinner	Salmon Poached with Vegetables	4.3
	Creamed Spinach	2.9
	Greens with Pecans & Blue Cheese	2.9
	Strawberry Mousse	2.7
	Total Net Carbohydrates	41.6

DAY THREE

		Net Carbohydrates
Breakfast	1/2 Baked Grapefruit	10.0
	Walnut Flax Muffin	2.4
	coffee, light cream	0.5
Snack	Slice of Walnut Pumpkin Loaf	4.2
	decaf coffee, light cream	0.5
Lunch	Egg Salad	10.0
	Easy Coleslaw	2.1
	sugar-free Jell-O	0.0
Snack	peach	7.1
Dinner	Cajun Pepper Steak	10.1
	Spinach & Strawberry Salad	4.5
	2 Icebox Cookies	4.0
Total Net Carbohydrates		55.4

DAY FOUR

		Net Carbohydrates
Breakfast	Sausage Pie	4.8
	Oatmeal Flax Muffin	4.1
	coffee, light cream	0.5
Snack	Citrus Protein Bar	4.5
	decaf coffee, light cream	0.5
Lunch	Spinach & Strawberry Salad	4.5
	1 ounce cheddar cheese	0.0
Snack	Oatmeal Flax Muffin	4.1
Dinner	Shepherd's Pie	5.9
	Summer Salad	6.3
	Quick & Easy Mousse	10.3
	Total Net Carbohydrates	45.5

DAY FIVE

		Net Carbohydrates
Breakfast	Eggs Benedict	4.7
	1/2 cup sliced strawberries	3.6
	coffee, light cream	0.5
Snack	Walnut Flax Muffin	2.4
	decaf coffee, light cream	0.5
Lunch	Salmon Avocado Salad	4.0
	Easy Coleslaw	2.1
	1/2 cup raspberries	2.9
Snack	Citrus Protein Bar	4.5
Dinner	Baked Balsamic Chicken	1.1
	Asparagus in Foil	3.5
	Zucchini Ribbons	4.4
	Oriental Coleslaw	4.8
	2 Almond Peanut Butter Cookies	2.3
	Total Net Carbohydrates	41.3

DAY SIX

		Net Carbohydrates
Breakfast	Sausage Pie	4.8
	Orange Cranberry Muffin	4.9
	coffee, light cream	0.5
Snack	Citrus Protein Bar	4.5
	decaf coffee, light cream	0.5
Lunch	Hearty Vegetable Soup	7.3
	1/2 cup blackberries	5.3
Snack	1/4 cup almonds	1.0
Dinner	Chicken Cacciatore	8.8
	Grapefruit & Spinach Salad	6.7
	1/2 cup raspberries	2.9
Total Net Carbohydrates		47.2

DAY SEVEN

		Net Carbohydrates
Breakfast	1/2 Baked Grapefruit	10.0
	Oatmeal Flax Muffin	4.1
	coffee, light cream	0.5
Snack	1/4 cup almonds	1.0
	decaf coffee, light cream	0.5
Lunch	Oriental Chicken Salad	11.6
	sugar-free Jell-O	0.0
Snack	2 sticks celery, 2 tbsp cream cheese	2.3
	herb tea	0.0
Dinner	Poached Salmon with Citrus Sauce	4.2
	Creamy Zucchini	3.7
	Asparagus in Foil	3.5
	Easy Coleslaw	2.1
	2 Flax Cookies	3.6
	Total Net Carbohydrates	47.1

Del and Colette: Comox, British Columbia

Hi Harv & Patricia:

Thank you for introducing us to a new way of life! It was meant to be that you would pull into the RV park in Blythe while we were there. I read your book before we left. We decided to give this a go and on April 15 I weighed in at 204. My goal was to try and reach 175, but guess what? At my weekly weigh-in this morning 172 flashed up on the scale. I can't believe how comfortable I feel — no more tight clothes and four notches less on the belt. I have encouraged quite a few people to try this new way of living and many are interested when I tell them how easy it is. Colette has dropped 15 pounds but can't exercise much as she is waiting for cartilage repair in her right knee. She looks and feels great and really likes trying on clothes two sizes smaller.

As you may recall, I have been troubled with IBS (irritable bowel syndrome) for 40 years — well, low and behold it is no more. That in itself is a real blessing as I'm sure you know.

We have tried lots of recipes and not a bad one in the bunch. We always have chocolate nut or citrus bars in our freezer. I don't know how many times I heard people say: "It's not the potato that is bad for you, it's what you put on it." How wrong they were. People can't believe we eat desserts with whipped cream! We are excited about the new us. Take care and keep up the good work.

SLOW CARB FOR SPECIAL NEEDS

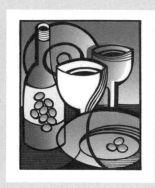

Slow Carb for Special Needs

We receive many questions on our Web site about the implications of the slow-carb approach for children and adolescents, for individuals with diabetes, food allergies, colon disorders, or for those who are vegan or vegetarian. We believe the recommendations we have made concerning nutrition can be adapted to suit any special dietary needs or audiences and have included some additional information for these people in the sections that follow.

Slow-Carb for Adolescents: Kid-Friendly Meals and Exercise

Recent articles in the media have alerted the public to the growing epidemic of overweight and obese children. From "fat farms" to special visits to the dietician to summer camps for big kids, one thing is clear: youth are facing severely compromised health and are at risk of early heart disease unless dramatic changes are made. The epidemic has been called "nothing short of a public health disaster." Overweight youth also suffer from feelings of insecurity, inadequacy, and low self-esteem, often worsened with the growing incidence of bullying in schools.

Maclean's magazine in its August 5, 2002, issue reported "33 percent of Canadian boys were overweight in 1996 — triple the rate in 1981 — while the number of overweight girls swelled to 27 percent from 13 percent. The ranks of these obese children-the kids in danger of getting adult-type diseases before they stop believing in Santa Claus — have soared even more dramatically: 10 percent of boys and 9 percent of girls are now considered obese. Visits to fast food restaurants in Canada ballooned by 200 percent between 1977 and 1995 as parents opted for handy, cheap (and fat laden) grub over the home cooked variety. And waistlines are thickening at home, too, as kids sit down to high sugar breakfast cereals and suck up bottles of pop in front of the TV. Suspicions are spreading that the low protein, high carbohydrate diet long favored by the health establishment may actually have contributed to obesity rates."

People magazine's November 4, 2002, issue reported, "Today juvenile obesity is rocking an escalating number of American households. According to a Center for

Disease Control and Prevention study released in October [2002] 15 percent of children between the ages of 6 and 19 are overweight or obese (double the number 20 years ago); so are 10 percent of 2- to 5-year-olds. With that surge has come a raft of related health problems. The estimated annual hospital tab for juvenile-obesity-related illnesses is $127 million."

The health risks for kids who are overweight or obese include many of those we associate with obese adults, except that they are manifest before the adolescents reach the age of 20. Adult onset diabetes is now called Type II Diabetes because of the large number of adolescents who are learning to live with its risks of heart disease, stroke, kidney failure, and problems with vision and circulation. The number of children with gallbladder disease has tripled in the past 20 years and the incidence of sleep-related breathing disruptions has skyrocketed. Being overweight puts youth at higher risk of heart attack, stroke, high blood pressure, and other chronic diseases normally seen only in adults.

Perhaps the most alarming statistics were presented at the February 2004 American College of Preventive Medicine Annual Meeting in the discussions of *The Obesity Epidemic: A Consequence of Our Success.* Dr. Sonia Caprio from the Yale University School of Medicine reported an increase in the rates of obesity in youth and an increase in the incidence of Type II Diabetes: "Among obese pre-adolescents, 24 percent have impaired glucose tolerance. Among obese adolescents, 20 percent have impaired glucose tolerance. Impaired glucose tolerance, or pre-diabetes, is an intermediate state between normal glucose tolerance and Type II Diabetes." Dr. Katz, also at the conference, cautioned that "in the future, children may have shorter life expectancies than their parents and could be more harmed by food than by tobacco, alcohol, and drug abuse combined. Because diabetes is an important cardiovascular risk factor, myocardial infarctions (heart attacks) could occur among adolescents within this decade."

A slow-carb approach is as effective and healthy for children as it is for adults, and recommendations for grams of carb intake are the same for adolescents as for adults — with some minor adaptations in order to make it more appealing for teens. If you have an adolescent in your home who is overweight or obese, the slow-carb approach will provide a healthy weight loss plan that is nutritionally balanced and will ensure that they have sufficient energy for daily activities while remaining alert in school. If you have other children in the house who do not need to lose weight, they should eat a maintenance level of carb intake rather than a weight loss level.

We recommend that adolescents who need to lose weight restrict their carbohydrate intake to between 40 and 70 grams a day with an average of 50 grams a day. This will allow one daily fruit serving, with plenty of vegetables, some whole grains, and protein. Finding the optimum level of slow-carb intake for your child will probably involve some trial and error over the course of a month. Most young people, even those with a sedentary lifestyle, have a higher rate of metabolism than adults, so an adolescent can eat more grams of carb per day than an adult and still achieve weight loss.

It is very important for kids to keep a Food Diary if they are going to achieve successful weight loss following the slow-carb plan. If the child is too young to accurately chart their food intake, then a parent or older sibling will have to assist them. We recommend a weekly weigh-in to track success and provide positive feedback to reinforce efforts. Your child did not become overweight in a day or a week so let them lose slowly and safely. A slow steady weight loss is more likely to feel less like a diet and encourage the behavioral changes that contribute to permanent healthy eating practices. It also allows your child to adapt to their new appearance, energy level, and physical abilities more gradually.

If you have an energetic child who needs to eat larger quantities of the slow-carb foods, it may be a matter of purchasing and preparing special foods that are appealing to avoid feelings of deprivation or hunger. Eventually, your children will learn to eat satisfying, tasty, and nutritious meals and still lose weight. Whatever you can do to make this switch easy and flexible will go a long way in improving the level of acceptance by your children.

Some children can be fussy eaters so you will need to be especially creative in your approach to meal planning. If your child has been eating high-carb and high-sugar foods, they'll need a few weeks to get over cravings and get used to the changes in their blood sugar so that they don't feel hungry all the time. Serve oatmeal with sliced strawberries or peaches and a little milk for breakfast. Regular oatmeal takes a few minutes to cook and has a low Glycemic Index (GI) (turns more slowly to blood sugar), while the instant variety is high glycemic. The cold cereal Vive from Kellogg's is soy-based (extra protein) and is an easy breakfast for kids. All Bran Extra Fiber has only 7 grams of net carb per half cup serving. Make some of the low-carb muffins with eggs or a baked grapefruit in the morning for lots of energy.

Be sure to include protein snacks throughout the day, such as low-carb muffins, cheese strings, nuts, seeds, trail mix (almonds, cashews, peanuts, a few raisins, and sunflower or pumpkin seeds). Be sure to use only a small number of raisins, as they are very high in sugar. Beef jerky or pork rinds are like potato chips with zero carbs. Pepperoni sticks or hard-boiled eggs are also good snacks. Pre-packaged sugar-free jelly desserts can be kept in the fridge along with a big bowl of sugar-free Jell-O, plain yogurt (or mixed with fresh fruit, nuts, and seeds), or celery sticks, cucumber slices, raw carrots, strawberries, peaches, or kiwi. Note that you will need to control the number of fruit servings per day during weight loss.

Lunches for school can be a challenge if your child insists on having a sandwich. Today there are many low-carb or whole grain breads available in specialty stores. Homemade low-carb bread is also an option — check out the recipes in the Recipes section of this book. You can send your child to school with an open-faced sandwich without any negative impact on their target for carb intake. Butter is a better option than margarine because most margarine is made by dehydrogenating or partially dehydrogenating the product, which converts the fat into a trans fatty acid. That said, some margarines on the market do not contain the hydrogenated fats. Make sure there is plenty of protein like chicken, fish, meat, eggs, or cheese to compensate. Roll-ups (see recipe) instead of sandwiches and slow-carb soups or chili in a thermos also work.

Include slow-carb fruit, sugar-free Jell-O, an easy mousse made with sugar-free pudding mixes, or a Lindt Rich Dark Chocolate bar (70 percent cocoa with very little sugar — this is a low glycemic chocolate with only 13 grams of carb for four big squares!) for something sweet. Breyers ice cream has recently launched a low-carb variety in a number of flavors including vanilla, chocolate, and strawberry. This low-carb ice cream has only four grams of net carb per half cup serving.

Other companies are selling frozen fudge and ice cream bars that have three to five grams of carb. The number of these treats ought to be kept to a minimum during weight loss as they can trigger cravings or cause a stall in weight loss if eaten too frequently. They also contain sugar alcohols that can have a laxative effect if taken in large quantities.

Water is the best drink, but you can also give your kids a diet pop or fruit drinks made with Splenda rather than aspartame, in lieu of regular fruit drinks or juice boxes in their lunch bag. These options will supply taste without carbs.

Exercise plays a significant role in weight loss for children. If you are in danger of raising a couch potato dedicated to computer games, chat rooms, and e-mail rather than 30 to 90 minutes a day (recommended by the Canadian Pediatric Society) playing street hockey, walking the dog, biking, hiking, swimming, basketball, volleyball, tennis, soccer, football, dancing, yoga, gymnastics, skiing, or running, then perhaps you need to initiate a family activity and lead by example.

It is important to be active enough to burn not only the food your children eat, but also the fat they have been storing. The more active your children become, the easier it gets and the more they will enjoy it. Exercising with a friend and being active within the constraints of your child's physical ability will improve his or her metabolism and make a big difference in attitude and appearance. Keep track of activity in the Food Diary and take exercise into account when charting weight loss and carb intake.

A study published in August 2003 in the *International Journal of Obesity* notes that "Playing the piano or taking an art class may not burn a lot of calories, but children can't eat if their hands are busy." The study also found that "Kids who ride bikes or play road hockey spend more hours on the move than those in sports leagues." It isn't necessary to invest time and money in organized sports to ensure that your kids are more active, but it is necessary to set targets and to help them find activities they enjoy.

Diabetics

Slow-carb living will not solve all the problems for diabetics, but it can improve the situation for some. Diabetics cannot produce enough insulin, so the carbohydrates that are converted to sugar cannot be adequately moved into the cells, and the body ends up with too much carbohydrate, in the form of sugar, in the blood. Controlling blood sugar levels can be a complicated balancing act. The diabetic is also at risk of getting too much insulin either because too much was injected, or because they didn't consume enough carbohydrate for the quantity injected. This imbalance between too much insulin and too little carbohydrate can lead to diabetic coma. Eating carbohydrates that convert slowly to blood sugar eliminates the spikes in demand for insulin and allows the pancreas to produce smaller amounts of insulin over longer periods of time. As a result, diabetics will usually find that once established on a slow-carb diet they can decrease the amount of insulin they inject or the amount of oral medication they need.

People with a family history of diabetes, especially if they are overweight, are at greater risk of diabetes than the general population. Women who developed gestational diabetes (temporary diabetes during pregnancy) are also at greater risk of developing Type II Diabetes later in life, particularly if they are overweight. Slow-carb living will help these people lose the extra weight and maintain a steady blood sugar level without stressing the pancreas. Both these changes will help keep the risk of Type II Diabetes to a minimum.

Digestive Disorders

We have had many readers write to us who suffer from digestive concerns and wonder whether a slow-carb approach would be of benefit to them. We caution them that digestive problems can have many causes, so they should consult their own doctor before embarking on a slow-carb eating plan. Of course if they are already under medical care for their problem, it is even more critical that any action they take is in consultation with their doctor. Many doctors are recommending a slow-carb diet to alleviate digestive problems such as irritable bowel syndrome (IBS) and colitis.

Cancer

It is beyond our scope to discuss the extensive medical research documenting the effects of diet on cancer, but a recent medical article dealing with slow-carb foods that reduce the Glycemic Load (GL) is of relevance here. An article in the *Journal of the National Cancer Institute* in 2002 stated that evidence from both animal and human studies suggests that abnormal blood sugar metabolism plays an important role in the cause of pancreatic cancer. The authors in this study investigated whether diets high in foods that rapidly increase blood sugar levels are associated with an increase of pancreatic cancer.

The findings come from the Nurses' Health Study that included 88,802 U.S. women and 180 case subjects with pancreatic cancer who were diagnosed during the 18-year follow-up. They calculated sucrose, fructose, and carbohydrate intakes using the Glycemic Index (GI) and concluded that a diet high in Glycemic Load (GL) may increase the risk of pancreatic cancer in women who have a pre-existing case of insulin resistance. The results of this study do not mean that diets high in carbohydrates cause all cancers, but rather suggest another benefit of adopting the slow-carb approach.

Food Allergies

Many people today have food allergies that cause stomach aches, headaches, and digestive disorders, while others may even risk their lives if they eat the wrong foods. Whatever your allergy, it is possible to eat slow-carb while taking your diet restrictions into consideration. A slow-carb approach can be especially effective for people who are either sensitive or allergic to wheat (celiac). Very few of our recipes use wheat in any form, and those that do use it in only small amounts. If you have celiac disease, ignore the recipes that use wheat and enjoy all the others. Many people who suffer from irritable bowel syndrome (IBS), colitis, and other digestive diseases find that they are able to reduce or eliminate their symptoms when they eat according to slow-carb recommendations. We suspect that more people actually have sensitivities to wheat than are aware of it.

We have heard from readers who suffer from headaches and mood swings, asking whether controlling carbohydrates would help alleviate these symptoms. In virtually every case, they report that reducing the level of carbohydrate intake has had dramatic positive results. We were interested to read in the *False Fat Diet* by Dr. Elson M. Haas that wheat is one of seven foods to which many people react. The other foods to which people often react adversely are dairy products, corn, sugar, eggs, soy, and peanuts. It is quite possible to be sensitive to foods without being truly allergic to them. So, although you do not go into shock when you eat these foods, you may experience symptoms like indigestion, bowel problems, headaches, sore throat, swollen glands, and others. Eating foods we are sensitive to stresses our immune system and weakens our response to stimuli such as pollens. Dr. Haas outlines an elimination diet to help you determine which foods you react to; cravings for a particular food can also be an indication of a sensitivity to it.

Individuals with lactose intolerance (sensitivity to the sugar in milk and other dairy products) also accommodate a slow-carb approach with little or no problem. Because there is less lactose in cream than in skim milk or 2 percent milk, those who are lactose intolerant are better off using light cream than whole milk. For those who are very intolerant, substitute soy milk products in recipes, but watch your numbers, as soy milk has higher carb content than cream. Low-carb protein shakes (read the label because many protein shakes are high in carbs) made with heavy cream, goat milk, or soy milk are also quick and tasty.

Those who are allergic to walnuts can use almonds or pecans as substitutes in recipes. This will change the taste slightly, as well as the carb content of the dish, but the change will not be significant. Flax seed meal or plain flax seed, ground sunflower or pumpkin seeds, ground sesame seeds or soy nuts, and soy flour or oat flour can also be substituted for ground nuts in recipes. These ingredients can be found in health food or grocery stores. The sunflower and pumpkin seeds will add a different flavor, as will the soy flour and the oat flour. Oat flour is a little higher in carb content, so you will want to be careful not to use too much. The flax seed tastes a bit like bran. The use of flax seed meal will add texture and lots of fiber to the recipe. Seeds can be used in the same quantities as nuts, but soy flour will have to be used in smaller quantities. Raisins can sometimes be substituted in baking, though this would bump up the carb content.

There are solutions to almost every dietary concern if you use a little imagination. If you have a question or concern about your special dietary requirements, visit us on the Web at www.slowcarbforlife.com and we will try to resolve your concerns.

Vegetarians

Many people refer to themselves as vegetarian when what they mean is they don't eat meat, or red meat, or they only eat chicken and vegetables, or they eat fish, chicken, and vegetables, or they eat eggs and cheese and vegetables, or any combination of the above. These dietary restrictions may mean that they will have to do some substituting of certain foods or ingredients in the recipes to suit preferences, but the effects should be the same. Vegetarians often rely heavily on the high-carb foods for filler in their meals, including large quantities of bread, rice, potatoes, and certain fruits. In order to get sufficient amounts of protein during your day we suggest substituting soy and soy products (including tofu), nuts, seeds, whole grains, and protein shakes and products made with protein powders. Chicken, fish, eggs, and cheese are also good protein sources but may be omitted depending on the nature of your vegetarianism.

As with all other foods, be sure to read the labels and count the correct number of carbs for the serving size that you have chosen. When manufacturers make many vegetarian products they replace the meat with grains, beans, legumes, and other high-carbs vegetable products. Pay particular attention to the labeling of vegetarian products to ensure you are not getting an unwanted carb load. It is always best to use these products in moderation and make your own from scratch whenever possible.

Vegans

Individuals who are vegan do not eat any animal products, including cheese, dairy products, or eggs. This level of restriction can make it more difficult to follow slow-carb, but with some imagination and planning it can be done. As with other vegetarian approaches, the biggest challenge here is to provide sufficient protein during the day. Many people who eat this way are very dependent upon grains, legumes, and beans for protein. Unfortunately, some of these foods tend to be high in carbohydrates. Tofu and tofu cheeses as well as other soy products contain good protein sources and can be substituted for meat, as can other lower carb vegetables. The following options will make it easier for vegans to adhere to the slow-carb plan.

- Substitute tofu in recipes to replace chicken.
- Eat lots of nuts and seeds in salads and as snacks.
- Choose legumes carefully as these are a little higher in carbs, but necessary for you to get enough protein.
- Eat whole-grain breads that are lower in carb content.
- For veggie stir-fries, try cooked, cut cabbage under the stir-fry instead of rice.
- Try the low-carb protein shakes for quick breakfasts and easy snacks.
- Add soy and whey protein in your baking and cooking.
- Use cooked cabbage in lieu of pasta.

Vitamin Supplements

Most traditional nutrition advisors maintain that if you follow their recommendations you don't need vitamin supplements, but this does not take into account the loss in nutrient value in our foods resulting from chemically stimulated growth, early harvest to accommodate lengthy distances of transport to market, the time of the transport, storage time in warehouses and on store shelves, and the delay between purchase and use. If the food is frozen it loses additional nutrients. Each step in the process takes some nutrient value out of the food.

Because of this, even if you manage to eat all the types and amounts of food recommended, you are likely to be deficient in some of the required nutrients. Furthermore, some of the nutrient value may not get absorbed because of medication you are taking, temporary ill health, or alcohol consumption. When all the factors are considered there is a very high likelihood that your body isn't getting all of the nutrients it needs for maximum health. The logical way to make up for these shortfalls is to add the missing nutrients in the form of supplements. Dietary supplementation is increasingly accepted, and even recommended, by dieticians, family doctors, and academics.

What should you take? The answer to that question depends on your age, gender, diet, and health status. For those who consider themselves to be in good health, with a reasonably healthy diet, we recommend that a standard store brand multivitamin, multi-mineral supplement, plus an additional 400 mg capsule of vitamin E, be taken daily. Make sure the brand you choose has at least 0.5 milligrams of folic acid. If you are not in full health, you ought to seek medical counsel for a prescription that specifically fits your needs.

Jacqueline: Toronto, Ontario

Patricia, your cookbook has helped me improve my overall health. I first purchased the book for a friend who needed to lose weight. Before I actually gave my friend the book, I began to read it myself, just out of curiosity. I have never had a weight problem, however I wondered what type of "diet tricks" this book boasted. To my delight, I learned that this book was not about "diet tricks." It was common sense eating, simple recipes that taste great, with ingredients that most of us have in our kitchens.

Not only were the recipes appealing, but when you discovered that by reducing your carbs you eliminated the symptoms of colitis I began to believe that perhaps I could be helped. I have suffered all my life from irritable bowel syndrome (IBS) and have never had much success in treating it. Because I didn't want to lose weight, I added fruit and extra portions to my meals, but I stayed away from the refined carbs. Since following this approach I have not suffered from IBS, except of course, when I cheat! Delighted with the results, I purchased another book for my friend. She and her husband both followed the advice in your book, and have both lost weight without feeling deprived. They are now, like me, true believers in this healthy eating lifestyle!

STRATEGIES FOR SUCCESS: TIPS AND SHORTCUTS

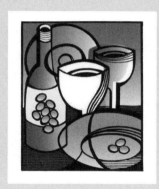

Strategies for Success: Tips and Shortcuts

Strategies to help you achieve your goals, including everything from developing your slow-carb grocery list, to knowing what to eat and drink when visiting with friends, to motivating yourself with healthy rewards, can make the whole program more manageable and more fun. A slow-carb program that is well thought out is as satisfying as eating high carb. Soon food cravings for potatoes, bread, and rice will disappear and you will focus instead on your positive results.

Change Your Eating Habits

Habits of any kind are difficult to change, but eating habits may be the most difficult. Examine when and why you eat. It would be simple if we all ate only when we were hungry and stopped eating when we felt full. Unfortunately, many of us eat out of boredom, out of habit, or to fill an emotional need. When you eat, are you usually alone or with friends or family? Is it at regular meal times or is it in the evening? Do you usually feel happy or sad when you eat? Maybe you feel lonely. For many of us, the evening is the most difficult time to stay away from food. During the day we are busy with school, work, or play, but in the evening we have time on our hands. We tend to be inactive after our evening meal and many of us sit at home and watch TV or read. If you snack too much (even with slow-carb snack foods you can have too much of a good thing) when you don't have anything to occupy your hands try stretching, knee bends, or walking on the spot, anything to divert your attention from food. If you know that you have a hard time staying away from the fridge at eight or nine o'clock in the evening, then go for a walk with the dog, the kids, your partner, or your neighbor instead. Do anything that gets you up and about and away from food. Change your routine.

Some of us eat if we are feeling under stress at work or home. The exertion of a walk, a golf game, a swim, a tennis match, or a yoga class will take your thoughts away from the stressor and will encourage the body to release endorphins, the body's natural feel better fix. Physical exertion can help you sleep better at night and has the additional benefit of burning extra calories. It may take some experimentation to find the activity that best suits your physical condition and your particular interests, but it is well worth the investment.

Revisit Your Goals

When you feel unmotivated to continue on the slow-carb plan, revisit your goals. Why did you decide to go on the plan in the first place? Did you want to lose the pounds that you put on over the past 10 years? Did you want to fit back into the clothes you wore when you were two sizes smaller? Did you want to be more physically active and achieve that sense of physical freedom that you had when you were slimmer? Did you want to reduce your blood pressure or your cholesterol? When you are tempted to eat something that is not part of your plan, remind yourself why you decided to change your habits.

Be Patient and Resolved

If you make a bad food choice or completely fall off the wagon and binge on pizza or some other high carb food, don't dwell on your slips or mistakes, think instead about all the positive steps you have taken. If you make a choice to eat some high-carb foods and want to do something about it, go for a long walk or involve yourself in some other form of physical activity. Forgive yourself and vow to try harder. This is a lifelong strategy and everyone has days that are easier than others.

Do It with a Buddy

Many people find it easier to stick to a change in eating habits if they have a buddy that they can confide in, work with, or with whom to exchange ideas and tips. Have slow-carb potluck dinners, go slow-carb shopping for new products, and develop slow-carb varieties of your favorite recipes. Even if your buddy is not following a slow-carb approach, someone to talk to about your successes and setbacks in person, over the phone, over the Internet, or by mail provides support and encouragement. This is one reason we decided to launch a Web site where people can go to ask us questions, to find new recipes, and to read about new research.

Read Labels

There is always someone in the aisle of the grocery store pouring over the small print on the label. We want you to become one of these people, especially when you first start your slow-carb plan. Take time with your shopping and read all of the salad dressing labels until you find one or two that appeal to your palate and have a low-carb content, rather than the low fat ones that are high in sugar and therefore higher in carbs. Vinaigrette dressings often have only a couple of grams of carb in each tablespoon and there are also creamy dressings that are very low carb. Pay attention to the serving size for which the nutrition information is being given. If you like a lot of dressing on your salad, you need to consider this in the calculation of your carb count. More and more manufacturers are catering both to the diabetic population and the low-carbers of the world, so low-sugar diabetic chocolates, jams and jellies, sugar-free hard candy, mints and gum, and a host of other products are being developed.

Watch Serving Sizes

It is important to pay attention to the serving sizes in the recipes as well as the serving sizes in commercial foods. If you have a large appetite, especially at the start of your slow-carb plan, it may be necessary to have more than a single serving of a dish. This is perfectly acceptable as long as you are increasing your carb count by the serving size you eat. You will find over time that the protein in your meals and the bulk of the vegetables should reduce your need for large servings, and will help you feel pleasantly full at the end of a meal.

Eat Breakfast

Statistics show that over 60 percent of the people who take weight off and keep it off eat breakfast every day. If you need to get up and make breakfast for other family members, or get to work, it is particularly important that you have all the ingredients available. If you get up and go to the gym before work, or if your job is physically demanding, you will want more protein than if you get up and go to the office and sit all day. Eating when you get up will also keep your body from going into starvation mode, hoarding calories because it is unsure when it will be fed again. A nutritional breakfast will keep your blood sugar at an even level for the morning. Even if you don't feel hungry when you get up, your body needs nourishment to get going again. When you skip breakfast you set yourself up for a dramatic swing in blood sugar which can negatively affect your energy and your ability to think, and will cause you to feel hungry. If you are driving to work, at the office, or on the golf course when this hunger hits you, it is likely that you may not have slow-carb options.

Drs. Eades in *The Protein Power Lifeplan* explain, "Studies have shown that what you (or your kids) eat for breakfast sets the tone of what you (or they) will want to eat at the end of the day. Recent studies have proven that a higher protein, higher fat breakfast, lower in sugars and starches, will prevent overeating later on and may be a big factor in preventing the rising epidemic of childhood and adolescent obesity, a problem that has doubled in the last 10 years!" (p. 361). If you want to eat cold cereals, it is critical to calculate how much of the carb is fiber. The low-carb granolas are very tasty, but we suspect that their carb count may be higher than advertised considering the contents. With any cereal, whether hot or cold, you must always add the carb content of your milk to get the actual total carb content.

BREAKFAST OPTIONS SUITABLE FOR WEIGHT LOSS

	Net Grams of Carbohydrates
bacon or sausage or ham and eggs *	1.2
1/2 cup 1 percent cottage cheese	4.0
with 1/2 cup sliced strawberries	3.6
1/2 cup whole plain yogurt	7.0
with 1/4 cup toasted seeds and nuts	2.0
1/2 cup ricotta cheese	3.0
with 1/4 fresh chopped tomato	2.9
Citrus Protein Bar	4.5
Chocolate Protein Nut Bar	6.4
Magic Muffin	2.5
Coconut Zucchini Muffin	4.9
Lemon Carrot Muffin	9.0
Walnut Flax Muffin	2.4
Oatmeal Pumpkin Muffin	4.6
Flax & Oat Muffin	8.2
Eggs Benedict	4.7
Breakfast Pie	4.7
Strawberry Smoothie	6.2
Mushroom & Cheese Omelet	3.4
Mushroom & Spinach Frittata	3.1
Easy Cheesy Quiche	4.2
Smoked salmon, raw onion, capers, and lemon juice	3.6
Low-carb protein shake	4–5

* Eggs may be fried, scrambled, poached, or boiled.

BREAKFAST OPTIONS SUITABLE FOR MAINTENANCE

	Net Grams of Carbohydrates
Bowl of hot oatmeal *	14.0
with light cream	2.0
Bowl of hot oatmeal	14.0
with 2–3 sliced strawberries and cream	13.5
1/2 fresh grapefruit	10.0
1/2 Warm Baked Grapefruit	10.0
2 slices Low-carb Bread	10.0
1/2 cup 1 percent fat cottage cheese	4.0
with 1/2 cup sliced strawberries	3.6
or 1/2 cup fresh raspberries	2.9
or 1/2 cup blackberries	5.3
or 1/2 cup blueberries	8.2
1/2 cup whole plain yogurt	5.0
with 1/2 cup sliced strawberries	3.6
or 1/2 cup fresh raspberries	2.9
or 1/2 cup blackberries	5.3
or 1/2 cup blueberries	8.2
Low-Carb Hash Browns	5.9
Low-Carb Granola	8.0
Orange Cranberry Muffins	4.9
All Bran Extra Fiber with light cream	9.0

* When making your oatmeal, be sure to use regular oats that take three to four minutes to cook, and not the instant variety. The chemical process that is used to make the oats "instant" dramatically changes the Glycemic Index (GI). While regular oats have a low GI, the instant variety has a high GI and is therefore not recommended. The grams of carbohydrate were calculated based on

1/3 cup of the raw oats, as per manufacturer's labeling. You may want to add some Splenda to sweeten your oatmeal or a little cinnamon or nutmeg. You may use any of the weight loss breakfast options during maintenance as well. If you are adventurous and like to eat unusual foods, you can eat anything within your carb target for breakfast.

Plan Your Meals

You will find that meal planning is especially important during the initial months. Whether you work outside the home or stay at home to work, whether you are a student or retired, you need to plan so that you don't get caught with only high-carb options when hungry. Menus and foods will vary depending on whether you are on weight loss or maintenance, and can be done on a daily or weekly basis if you are organized. Proper meal planning may also help lower the cost of food as there will be less waste and better use of leftover foods. Take into account the slow-carb foods that are in season or on sale, and be flexible. If you walk around the perimeter of the store, you will usually find the fresh fruit, fresh vegetables, meat, fish, poultry, dairy products, eggs, and more. In the centre of the store you may want to pick up some sugar-free Jell-O and Splenda, but you are no longer interested in all the pre-packaged foods. To save time and money you may want to buy some frozen fruit or vegetables, but be sure they are slow-carb and do not contain added sugar. Determine which proteins you will eat over the next two or three days and freeze the other protein for later in the week.

Planning for lunch is easier if you cook more protein for dinner than you'll eat. Whether you eat lunch at home, at work, or at play, cooked protein is a quick and easy lunch to accompany salad or coleslaw, or cheese or nuts to round out your meal. In cold weather when you want something hot for lunch, reheat meals frozen in individual portions.

Your evening meal will likely be your main meal of the day, so pay attention to portion size and eat relatively early in the evening to allow your food to digest before bed. Lean muscle continues to burn small amounts of energy, even during sleep, so your body becomes slimmer. As you increase the amount of lean muscle tissue and decrease the adipose or fat tissue, you will become a more efficient energy burner, even in your sleep. An evening meal might typically contain a small salad or soup, a protein portion (fish, poultry, or lean meat), and two cooked vegetables with fruit or other slow-carb dessert. Finish your meal with either decaf coffee or herb tea.

There are many diets that admonish you for eating outside the meal plans that are prescribed, but it is unhealthy to allow yourself to become extremely hungry in between meals. How often do you make good food choices when you are starving? We believe it is more reasonable, in fact essential, to build some snacks into your meal plan to maintain a constant blood sugar (energy) level throughout the day, or for an energy boost in periods of heavier activity. If you have a longer than normal time between meals, you may need a snack to tide you over, or if you work in an environment where your co-workers take a coffee break together and have something to eat or drink, you will want to join them without sabotaging your weight loss. Remember to include your snacks in your daily Food Diary so you are being as accurate as possible with your carb count.

It is important that you eat until you are satisfied. If at the end of the meal you still feel hungry, additional salad or more vegetables will help fill you up. Your vegetable servings may be quite large at the beginning, but gradually should be reduced in size as you grow accustomed to the slow-carb lifestyle.

Few of us have the luxury of being able to spend an hour preparing dinner every evening, enjoying the quiet in the kitchen and the scents of fresh herbs being chopped or garlic sizzling. Most of us like to cook when we are rested and have plenty of time so we are not under any pressure. Those days are few and far between, however, so here are some strategies to make slow-carb cooking easier and faster.

Buy Fresh

Buy fresh meats, poultry, and fish, once weekly. Freeze anything you'll eat later in the week or put it directly into a zip-lock bag and add marinade. Give the bag a shake or two and then freeze. The poultry or meat will tenderize and flavor while it thaws and will be ready to cook (substitute dried herbs instead of the fresh herbs when freezing). Divide extra cooked servings into individual portions and either cube or slice it very thinly for freezing. Use it later for lunches, snacks, or to add to a salad or to a few cooked vegetables for a quick and easy meal. If you bake or poach salmon use the extra for salmon salad or cold salmon with a green salad. A rotisserie (barbecue) chicken with a green salad makes a great no fuss meal, and leftovers can make a chicken salad the next day or be made into soups, salads, or other quick meals. Save the carcass and freeze it to make your own chicken broth with onion, celery tops, carrot, dried herbs, and salt and pepper. Let this simmer for three to four hours (or all day) on the stove and then strain. Beef stock can be made with beef bones the same way and can be used as the base for homemade soups or in sauces. Freeze them in small individual containers. Egg whites freeze well, two to a freezer bag. These are available anytime for an omelet, scrambled eggs, or other dish that uses egg whites. Use cooked spaghetti squash instead of pasta and cover with your favorite tomato or meat sauce.

Substitute

Cabbage can be eaten raw or cooked and contains dietary fiber as well as vitamins and minerals. It has almost no carbs, and very few calories, so it is a perfect addition to many meals. Use raw cabbage in coleslaw of various types and in salads to add bulk and texture. Cut cabbage into thin strips, boil, and then add to a plate half full of whole-wheat pasta; you can have a full plate of pasta this way, with only half the normal carbs. Use it to replace rice under a stir-fry or a curry dish, or add to almost any soup to add bulk and flavor.

Coleslaw keeps well even when dressed, so you can make a big batch and keep it in the fridge until you need it. It is a great addition to any summer lunch, dinner, picnic, or barbecue. Add sunflower seeds (either raw or roasted), green or red grapes cut in half, small pieces of apple, or a few raisins to add color, flavor, and texture. Be careful with the raisins and apples so you don't add too many, as they are higher in carbs.

Use thinly sliced zucchini or eggplant in place of noodles for lasagna. Shredded zucchini can be used as slow-carb filler in many dishes, including meat loaf or cabbage rolls. Zucchini is very mild in flavor and will not overpower the rest of the dish if used appropriately. It can also be used as an ingredient in muffins and cookies.

A lettuce wrap is like a wrap without the bread. Package the ingredients separately if making the night before and allow your kids to put it together at lunch the next day. Leftover meat or chicken from dinner makes great wraps with lettuce, cheese, and a few tomato slices.

There is no need to give up things like cheese or pâté before a meal or just as a snack, but instead of crackers, cut slices of cucumber or zucchini to put them on. Some tuna with a little mayo and lemon juice served on cucumber or zucchini thins, or cream cheese or peanut butter on a celery stick are tasty slow-carb alternatives to keep you on track. For quick snacks or lunches visit the deli section of your local grocery store. This is a little more expensive than making your own salads or protein, but very convenient. Stick to green salads, coleslaw, veggie or spinach salads, cheese, and deli meats or chicken as good slow-carb choices.

Frozen mixed vegetables are easy to microwave or boil and work well in a quick stir-fry. We suggest you still use fresh produce as often as you can, but this gives you an option when time is tight or if you have come to the end of the money before the end of the month.

Think Ahead

Make up a big bowl of sugar-free Jell-O (labeled Light Jell-O in Canada) and keep it covered in the fridge for dessert or snacks during weight loss. You can whip up a small amount of heavy (whipping) cream with Splenda to serve with it.

If you can spend some time cooking on the weekends, it is easy to freeze foods like chili or homemade soups into individual servings. These make great lunches at home, in the office, or at school. Make a pot roast and freeze individual servings for later in the week. Make some low-carb muffins on the weekend and put them in the freezer to be taken out for breakfast, snacks, or lunches. If you are serving salads for lunch use a smaller (lunch sized) plate so there is not a lot of empty space.

Stick to the Plan When Eating Out

When we eat at home, it is easy for all of us to control our food intake. It is somewhat more difficult, but not impossible when eating out — either at the home of friends or in restaurants. Eating at a friend's can be more difficult than eating in a restaurant where there are many selections to choose from and an eager waiter who wants to keep you happy. You may want to mention to your host that you need to avoid certain foods to which you are allergic, have a sensitivity, or which you cannot eat due to a "health issue." This may be a slight overstatement, but an allergy to wheat will eliminate pasta as a main course, as well as bread and many high-carb desserts. When you advise people that there is a health issue involved in your eating preferences, they tend to be much more supportive and willing to do whatever they can to help. People will generally be more supportive of a health issue than if you tell them you are on a diet. It is also helpful if you are able to provide some options when people ask, "What do you eat?"

Another strategy, when guests in someone else's home, is to eat very small portions of the foods that are not slow-carb. It is not going to harm your food plan or make a dramatic change in the results you seek if you occasionally eat something outside your normal choice, provided your food intake for the next few days is adjusted to accommodate this indulgence. This is especially true during maintenance when your carb intake allows more flexibility. The other thing you can do is offer to bring a dish, a slow-carb dessert, appetizer, or a special salad that guarantees you can have your fill without worrying about the carb content.

Eating in restaurants is also easy if you have a few tricks up your sleeve. Ask your server not to bring a bread basket to the table, decline a potato, pasta, or rice, and ask if you might have a few extra vegetables on your plate instead. Many low-carb diets avoid any food that has been breaded, battered, and then fried, though our experience has not supported the claim that this encourages old cravings for high-carb food. Order fish and chips or chicken fingers without the chips and ask for additional coleslaw or salad instead. The hydrogenated fats that are used in deep-frying mean this should be a rare indulgence but once you are on a maintenance level of carb intake, you can experiment.

Take Slow Carb on the Road

Maintaining your slow-carb meal plan while traveling is more difficult than while at home where you control your food. Whether you are traveling in your own recreational vehicle, driving and staying in hotels, flying, or staying with friends, these travel tips should help you deal with each situation.

A camping trip or vacation in your own recreational vehicle, whether it is a large motor home or a small tent trailer, will be the easiest type of travel to allow you to maintain your food plan. You can grill hamburgers, chicken, fish, hot dogs, or other meat (no bun) and eat them with cheese, some fried onions and mushrooms, and a nice big salad. Bring extra salad makings, some coleslaw, and other raw vegetables for snacks and to fill in the meals, as well as slow-carb fruits or desserts. Have bacon and eggs for breakfast, or bake homemade low-carb bars or muffins and pack them with you. If you really want to have something outside your normal meal plan because you are on vacation, go ahead, but be warned that just one ice cream cone a day will put on weight.

If you are flying, whether for business or pleasure, on a four- to eight-hour flight you can hope that the meal served on board has sufficient slow-carb food (most in-flight meals are full of bread, cakes, cookies, and sandwiches) or you can be proactive. If the airline is serving a dinner that includes a chicken breast with vegetables and a small salad, you can ignore the bread and dessert on the tray and enjoy a healthy meal. Another option is to request a special meal. Most airlines allow passengers with special dietary needs to order meals. There are many options available from vegetarian, to gluten-free (no wheat products), to vegan (no dairy, meat, or eggs). Otherwise pack some snack foods in your carry-on luggage — a couple of low-carb bars, some almonds, grapes, and cheese — and stay hydrated with bottled water, soda water, tea, or diet drinks.

Following your slow-carb food plan while traveling by car and staying in hotels is easy with protein powder, a small plastic cup with a tight rubber lid, and some water. Shake well and *voilà*, you now have a chocolate or strawberry protein shake for breakfast. You don't have to leave your hotel room to find breakfast it takes five minutes, and you have three grams of carb and 20 to 25 grams of protein. If you go out, ask for your bacon and eggs or sausage and eggs to be served without the potato and bread. This avoids waste and ensures you aren't tempted to eat something you shouldn't.

If all you can find is fast food spots lining the highway, pick one that serves salads as an option or has a salad bar. Avoid croutons or Chinese noodles and choose a vinaigrette to avoid sugar in the dressing. Low-carb burgers, omelets, and other items on the slow-carb meal plan are also ideal. Keep bottled water or soda water in the car, and carry nuts in zip-lock bags and low-carb protein bars for snacks while you drive. Sugar-free hard candies, mints, and gum keep your mind off other high carb-snacks between meals.

If your trip is more than a week or two, find a department store with a scale and weigh-in, or find a scale in a drugstore that will give you your weight for a small fee. If you are staying with friends, you might ask if they have a scale you can use. It can be very reassuring when you are traveling to realize that you are maintaining your slow-carb program; it can also allow you to make adjustments in your food intake sooner rather than later.

Eating while staying with friends when you are on vacation can be a little more difficult than staying in hotels where you can choose your foods from a restaurant menu. Provide advance notice of your dietary peculiarities so your friends are not caught off guard. Tell your friends that they should feel free to serve bread and potatoes if that is their normal habit, but that you would prefer not to have these items on your plate. It can be a challenge to maintain your food preferences without being difficult guests. Travel with your protein powder so if normal breakfast options are all high carb, you can make a protein shake. Offer to help with the cooking or to cook a couple of slow-carb meals. If your friends are making every effort to serve food that you can eat but their ingredients are adding up to extra pounds, be candid with them. If you mention possible food allergies or benefits such as reduction in blood pressure or cholesterol, they may be more accommodating.

Give Yourself the Gift of Health for the Holidays

Holidays can be a stressful time for anyone, and fear of putting on weight when we indulge in a tendency to party too much, eat too much, and spend too much money just adds to our stress. How many people do you know who plan to put weight on during the holidays and then diet in the new year? Many social events involve food; the trick is to think about how you are going to approach your eating in advance of the event. If a buffet is served, it is usually easy to find enough foods of the slow-carb variety, but if you are worried about it have a slow-carb snack before leaving home to ensure that you are not too hungry when you arrive. Raw vegetables, stuffed mushrooms, nuts, and other slow-carb appetizers are fine. You will almost always find some slow-carb vegetables and a variety of salads, so load up on these foods so that your plate doesn't look empty.

Perhaps the biggest challenge during the holidays will be to resist all the desserts. Instead, eat fresh fruit or offer to bring a slow-carb Raspberry Cheesecake and a Chocolate Mint Cake to serve to the guests — they're delicious. For Christmas dinner choose to eat the turkey with some slow-carb cranberry sauce, a little gravy, and lots of vegetables. Do not eat the potato, sweet potato, or the turkey stuffing (see the recipe for slow-carb turkey stuffing). If you want to avoid drinking too much alcohol, take a large bottle of soda water. Eggnog is very high in carbs as is mulled wine, hot mulled cider, and fruit punch.

Here are some holiday hints to help you:

- Decide early whether you are going to adhere to your slow-carb regime or indulge a little.
- Eat all things in moderation.
- Keep your portions small.
- Offer to bring a dish or dessert.
- Have a slow-carb snack of your own before leaving.
- Eat raw veggies with dips, stuffed mushrooms, cheeses, salmon, or other fish dish.

- Avoid anything in pastry or with bread. Fill up on nuts.
- Limit your drinking to wine or hard liquor without regular soft drinks as mix.
- Avoid eating the mashed potatoes or stuffing and have an otherwise traditional meal.
- Make your own homemade slow-carb cranberry sauce, and substitute soy flour in the gravy.
- Serve Raspberry Cheesecake instead of high-carb desserts.

We have developed some menu options for entertaining so that your guests will enjoy the selections without even knowing they are eating slow-carb (unless you tell them)!

Meal Plans for Entertaining

HOLIDAY

		Net Carbohydrates
Brunch	Baked Grapefruit	10.0
	Eggs Benedict	4.7
	Walnut Flax Muffin	2.4
	Coffee with light cream	0.5
Snacks	Spicy Southern Pecans	1.3
	Cheese & Salmon Ball with cucumbers & celery	2.0
Dinner	Turkey	0.0
	Turkey Stuffing	4.1
	Cranberry Sauce	2.3
	Gravy	2.0
	Creamy Garlic Cauliflower	3.0
	Steamed green beans	2.9
	Puréed Turnip & Turnip	7.4
	Raspberries & Cream	10.0
	Decaf coffee with light cream	0.5
Total Net Carbohydrates		**53.1**

BRUNCH

	Net Carbohydrates
Mushroom & Spinach Frittata	3.1
sliced smoked salmon or	0.0
sliced cold ham	0.0
Oriental Coleslaw	4.8
1/2 cup sliced strawberries	3.6
Walnut Flax Muffin	2.4
decaf coffee, light cream	0.5
Total Net Carbohydrates	14.4

LUNCH BUFFET

	Net Carbohydrates
Chicken Salad	1.2
Cold Salmon with Dill Sauce	1.1
Grapefruit & Spinach Salad	3.4
Broccoli Salad	3.1

The carb count has been reduced by 50 percent for each serving to accommodate a less than full portion.

Total Net Carbohydrates	8.8

DINNER

OPTION #1

	Net Carbohydrates
Greens with Pecans and Blue Cheese	2.9
Salmon Poached with Citrus Sauce	4.2
Asparagus in Foil	3.5
Grilled Eggplant	4.9
Almond Carrot Cake	5.6
with Vanilla Custard Sauce	2.3
tea, decaf coffee	0.5
Total Net Carbohydrates	23.9

OPTION #2

	Net Carbohydrates
Salmon & Avocado Salad	4.0
Pot Roast	7.4
Asparagus in Foil	3.5
Julie's Middle Eastern Orange Cake	6.7
Total Net Carbohydrates	21.6

OPTION #3

	Net Carbohydrates
Spinach & Strawberry Salad	4.5
Chicken with Citrus Cranberry Sauce	4.3
Creamy Garlic Cauliflower	3.0
steamed green beans	2.5
Lemon Cream Pie	6.3
Total Net Carbohydrates	20.6

Rules for Slow-Carb Living

- Decide what your goal is and make sure it is achievable.
- Write it down and post it on your fridge or carry it in your wallet.
- Find a buddy and support each other by meeting at least once a week (over the phone or via e-mail if unable to meet face to face) to discuss your successes and setbacks.
- Get yourself a good low-carb cookbook.
- If you do decide to eat or drink something high in carbs, keep portions small.
- Offer to bring a dish or dessert if you are invited out to dinner.
- Eat three meals and three snacks (that contain protein) each day.
- Avoid feeling starved when you sit down to eat a meal.
- If you go to a restaurant for dinner, ask the waiter not to bring a bread basket to your table.
- If you sweeten your tea or coffee, use Splenda.
- Limit your drinking to wine and have only one glass.
- Walk 20 minutes each day.
- Keep a Food Diary and weigh yourself once weekly.

Cally: Brockville, Ontario

I have started week nine on maintenance today and because of post-holiday vigilance and renewed exercise activity I am down a couple of pounds from the ideal weight I have been maintaining. Quite unbelievable for one who has usually put on 8 to 10 pounds over the holidays! I have not been able to get into a size 10 since my girls were born, almost 30 years ago, and I still think I will wake up from a dream and bulge into my new clothes! No way! I'm so grateful to have stumbled onto your book and ideas and now have the knowledge and power to control how I feel and look. After my trip in October with regular-eating-friends, my friend who had watched and helped me figure out carb values for some of my recipes decided to give this way of eating a try. Since October she has shed 13 pounds but slipped on a couple over the holidays.

FREQUENTLY
ASKED QUESTIONS

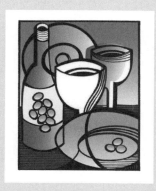

Frequently Asked Questions

We continue to receive emails and questions from readers at book signings or during radio or television call-ins, and as you might expect many of the same questions arise. There are detailed answers to most of these in the body of the book, but here are the most common questions and their abridged answers for quick reference.

What can I eat for breakfast?

Your options will vary depending on whether you are on weight loss or maintenance. We suggest eggs — fry them, scramble them, poach them, boil them, eat them with bacon or ham or sausage, add some tomatoes or hot sauce, make an omelet, cook a frittata. . . . Dr. Michael Mogadam, an assistant professor of medicine at Georgetown University in Washington, D.C., is a cholesterol disorders specialist who responded to a question in *Shape* magazine (June 2002) about whether the reader should eat egg whites only to cut down on cholesterol, as she eats eggs two or three mornings a week for protein. Mogadam says, "The beauty of the egg is in the yolk. The white has nothing but protein. The yolk has the nutrients, including vitamins, minerals, and antioxidants. Sure, the yolk also contains the fat and cholesterol. However, of the 6 grams of fat in a large egg, only 2 grams are saturated (bad fat). The other 4 are unsaturated and actually coronary friendly. What's more, 1 gram of the saturated fat is stearic acid, which behaves like monounsaturated fat (good fat). The bottom line: Only 1 gram of the 6 is the unhealthy kind. The other 5 grams of healthy fat more than offset this one gram. The cholesterol — about 213 milligrams per egg — is nothing to worry about either. The human body only absorbs 10-30 percent of that. Also, in most people, dietary cholesterol intake has a negligible effect on blood cholesterol levels. Research suggests that eating two eggs a day for 12 weeks raises LDL cholesterol by only 4 points, and the numbers level off soon thereafter. Over the years, it becomes a non-issue. The body adjusts. What does elevate blood cholesterol significantly is high intake of saturated fat (found in whole milk, cheese, and fatty red meat) and trans fat (found in cakes, cookies, and other commercial baked goods). One egg contains about 75 calories and 6 grams of protein. If you toss out the yolk, you lose 4.5 grams of protein and 59 calories, along with the vitamins A and D and folic acid."

You might also choose cottage cheese or whole plain yogurt with small toppings of fruit or nuts and seeds. For cereal try All Bran Extra Fiber or Vive or oatmeal (regular, not instant) with fresh fruit. Add low-carb protein powder for sustenance, like a Strawberry Smoothie, or slow-carb muffins. If you are comfortable with less traditional breakfasts, try a vegetable stir-fry or a green salad with nuts or tuna for protein. Almost anything is an option, keeping in mind the carbohydrate content and your daily target.

How is your plan different from that of Dr. Atkins?

We don't recommend you reduce your carbs to levels as low as Atkins, we don't protein load, and we eat a much more balanced diet (including fruit) during weight loss and especially once we are on maintenance. This as a lifestyle change, not a diet, so it has to be easy and it has to be for life.

Does eating slow-carb mean that I have to give up bread forever?

There are now many low-carb breads (three to six grams per slice) on the market and we've included recipes using whole grain products that you can bake at home. These should still be rare treats during your weight loss period. Read the labels to learn the grams of carb per slice as some manufacturers may be exaggerating the net carb content of their products. Experiment slowly and cautiously to track how your body responds to these products.

Do I have to completely give up potatoes, rice, and pasta?

These products should not be eaten during the weight loss phase of the slow-carb approach. Only you can determine what you want to gradually reintroduce into your meal plan as you adapt to a maintenance level. Keep in mind that a medium baked potato with skin has 51 grams of carbohydrate and virtually no nutritional value. If you feel you want to reintroduce some of these products into your meal plan, try brown rice (23 grams of carb per ½ cup, cooked) or whole-wheat pasta (19 grams of carb per ½ cup). Go slowly at first, don't try more than one of these products a week, while you record your intake and monitor your weight. Also pay attention to your body as it deals with these products. If you experience any indigestion, diarrhea, headache, or other symptoms, then you are better off eliminating these foods from your diet.

What does it mean when a label says "Net Carbs"?

Manufacturers prefer to advertise as few carbs as possible. In the past they simply didn't include the carbs in fiber or sugar alcohols (like maltitol) or glycerine because most people don't absorb these ingredients, they don't impact the blood sugar. A few years ago the U.S. FDA directed that all of these ingredients had to be included in the total carb count. Manufacturers now give you the net carb count where they subtract the fiber, sugar alcohols, and glycerine from the total carbs. You need to count only the net carbs in your daily intake.

Why do you recommend Splenda as a sweetener?

Splenda is a sugar substitute. It is a natural product with no known health risks. Unlike saccharin or aspartame, it has no chemical additives. It has no aftertaste and remains stable when heated so is excellent for cooking and baking. You will find it in the sugar aisle of any major grocery store.

How much weight can I expect to lose in an average week?

When you start your slow-carb weight loss plan, you may lose as many as five to seven pounds in the first week. Some of this will be fluid loss as your body adjusts to this approach to food, and as your metabolism switches to fat burning as a mechanism to produce energy. After this initial loss, you will lose anywhere from one to four pounds a week, on average. This average will vary with your level of carb intake, your weight, your activity level, and your natural metabolism. We recommend that you aim for one to two and a half pounds per week.

Is it true that a slow-carb diet can reduce my cholesterol?

Research shows that a low-carb diet is effective in lowering cholesterol, triglycerides, and blood pressure. Surprisingly, while following a slow-carb diet it is possible to add fat to your diet and still achieve these reductions. This is probably related to the insulin mechanism explained in Understanding Fats, and why many of the recipes have small amounts of fat in them. In fact, we intentionally increase the good fats in our diet.

If I go on a slow-carb diet, can I stop my cholesterol medication?

It is important to continue to follow your doctor's advice and stay on your medication. Almost everybody experiences a decrease in their total cholesterol level if they follow a slow-carb diet. What is even better is that the diet tends to increase the HDL cholesterol (the good stuff) and decreases the LDL cholesterol (the bad stuff). Triglycerides are also likely to go down and many people see a reduction in their blood pressure. You may want to have your doctor check your blood levels after several weeks (at least eight) on the program to see what effect it has had on you.

What would cause a stall in weight loss?

Most people who temporarily cease to lose weight (or stall) don't keep a Food Diary. If you aren't doing that, we strongly recommend that you start. It feels like a chore at the beginning, but after a week or two you become familiar enough with the carb content of the foods you eat regularly that it is easy to keep track. Furthermore, count the carbs in everything. It is tempting (and easy) to just ignore the few grams of carb in a glass of milk, or a few nuts, or a handful of berries, but when you write them down, they add up. Also, if you drink more than a couple of cups of regular coffee per day, it may be contributing to your stall, so substitute decaf to eliminate that problem. Watch that high-fiber cereals are low-carb. Many people do not tolerate the commercial low-carb bars in any quantity without either stalling or putting on some weight. We would suggest you cut these out first. Foods with a high salt content such as salted nuts, seeds, pork rinds, and other snack foods are often culprits, as are foods containing artificial sweeteners.

How do I get out of a stall?

Your body is making a significant adjustment to how it handles the food you eat and may take longer to adapt than you'd like. This period is called a plateau and is what you are interpreting as a stall. Usually if you persevere your body will adjust and you will lose weight again. If you persist for at least four weeks without any weight loss, then you need to change something. Start by doing a review of your Food Diary. Eliminate the causes noted above or try a process of trial and error. Are you getting enough exercise? If not, try adding a 30-minute walk on a daily basis. Are you snacking in the evening? Try some sugar-free Jell-O as a snack or sugar-free gum to avoid other snacks before bed. You may need to reduce your daily carb intake to kick-start the process. Add some vegetables (the slow-carb type) and salads to help fill your tummy and add bulk to your meals and just be patient, you body will work out the best balance for you.

Is it safe for my children to follow a slow-carb lifestyle?

Following a slow-carb lifestyle is healthy for anyone, including children, as long as they don't have a medical condition that complicates this. Shop for slow-carb varieties of breads and crackers, or use cucumber or zucchini instead of crackers. Initially this will be foreign, but if you are enthusiastic and lead by example most children seem quite willing to make the shift.

Will the medication I am taking affect the success of my weight loss program?

Most medications act by influencing the body's metabolism in some way. Your slow-carb eating program also influences metabolism so the short answer is yes. If you are taking any prescribed medication you should seek guidance from your family physician before you start your slow-carb program. See our reference list for some bedside reading on the subject.

What if I want to splurge and have a pizza one night?

Remember that this is your program. You can make whatever choices you feel are best for you. Pizza has somewhere between 20 and 60 grams of carb per slice so if you splurge, adjust your carbohydrate intake for the balance of the week to maintain your daily average. But be careful; if you indulge in this type of food, you may set yourself up for additional urges that might take you off track.

Can I eat Chinese food?

Be careful to choose vegetable dishes and dishes like cashew chicken and beef with broccoli that are not battered and deep-fried. Stay away from the sweet and sour dishes as they will have lots of sugar and the meats will be battered and deep-fried.

What do you do when you go to dinner at a restaurant?

We order a small green salad or soup to start and ask our server not to bring a bread basket to our table, so it doesn't tempt us and it doesn't go to waste. We order whatever we have chosen for our main meal, and ask that additional vegetables be substituted for potato or rice. We order fresh fruit for dessert as well as tea or decaf coffee.

What are the high-carb foods I should avoid?

The foods that are high in carbs include white breads, baked goods, pasta, potatoes, white rice, and anything with sugar. High-carb vegetables include peas, corn, and beets. All fruits have natural sugars called fructose but those with a high carbohydrate content include bananas, apples, grapes, oranges, pears, and raisins. Look up your favorite foods in the Carb Counter to become familiar with the carb content of each.

What are the low-carb foods?

Low-carb foods include most proteins (eggs, cheeses, fish, poultry, meat, and nuts) as well as certain low-carb vegetables such as lettuce, celery, cucumber, mushrooms, sprouts, cauliflower, broccoli, green beans, asparagus, and cabbage. Some fruits are lower in carb than others, including strawberries, raspberries, blackberries, blueberries, watermelon, kiwi, pineapple, and peaches.

I am a diabetic; is it safe for me to follow a slow-carb diet?

A slow-carb diet is an excellent way to help manage diabetes since it helps control the blood sugar and therefore the insulin demand. Most people who switch to slow-carb are able to keep their blood sugars normal while on the diet. We have heard from many readers, including insulin-dependent diabetics, who have been able to reduce their medication after following a slow-carb diet. However, you should not do this without consulting your doctor. Many physicians and dieticians are now recommending low-carb diets to their diabetic patients.

I am a vegetarian. Can I follow a low-carb lifestyle?

We have many readers who are vegetarian, including a fair number who are vegan. It is certainly possible to live a healthy slow-carb lifestyle as either. Obviously the more strictly you follow a vegetarian diet, the greater the challenge getting the protein you need, but don't make the mistake of forgetting to count the carbs in the vegetarian foods you use for protein. Eat lots of fish and substitute tofu for many of the chicken dishes, use more nuts and seeds in salads and for snacks, and eat legumes (higher in carbs, but a good source of protein). Use lots of soy and whey protein in your baking and cooking and try out the protein shakes we recommend for quick breakfasts and easy snacks. If you want to keep some bread in your diet, try the new low-carb varieties, or the sprouted grain breads that are lower carb. If you do veggie stir-fries, try cooked, cut cabbage under the stir-fry instead of rice. Do the same for pasta.

Are there any medical conditions that preclude a slow-carb lifestyle?

There is virtually no medical condition that would prevent you from living a slow-carb lifestyle. That said, if you have a medical condition you should consult your family doctor before you begin a slow-carb program.

I have been on the slow-carb diet for two weeks and I am constipated. What can I do?

Having some constipation in the early stages of eating slow-carb is a common side effect. It usually abates, but in the meantime eat high-fiber vegetables such as cabbage, cauliflower, or broccoli, and try Kellogg's All Bran Extra Fiber. Try sprinkling flax seed meal on your food (salads are a good option) or eat flax muffins. If you are on maintenance, try some fruit in the morning. If you are on weight loss you should probably stick to berries because they are fairly low in carbs and can also improve digestion.

How important is exercise in my slow-carb lifestyle program?

Exercising is an important component in achieving your maximum health. Adopting a regular exercise routine could mean walking for 20 minutes at noon or after dinner or taking up yoga, biking to work, or doing Tai Chi in the park. Find something fun that motivates you and raises your heart rate so that the pounds you shed will take extra stress off your body and make the whole process easier.

If you have a question that wasn't answered here, we invite you to ask us through our Web site at www.slowcarbforlife.com.

Joanne: Turner Valley, Alberta

Dear Patricia,

Thank you for getting back to me so quickly re my cry for help about my eight-year-old. I used all your suggestions and now a month into our new way of eating our family has lost a total of 49 pounds. My husband has lost 13 pounds, my 11-year-old daughter has lost 10 pounds, my 8-year-old son has lost nine, and I have lost 17. Thank you so much.

We do seem to need one meal a week of cheating. Last week they begged me for spaghetti but they ate only half of what they would have usually eaten. My son is no longer begging for food every 15 minutes, my daughter is becoming more confident in her appearance, and I have stayed on this for more than two weeks (my usual breaking point). It is so much easier cooking for the whole family than just for me. The recipes are wonderful. They all love them, and I have started to enjoy cooking again. (Mainly due to the fact that my family loves the recipes.) We make a big deal of supper — a nicely set table, good manners, no one leaves until everyone is done. It is sometimes hard to pull off, but we seem to make it six out of seven days.

I did have to make a few changes. We probably are eating more fruit than what you would recommend and because of children's tastes my vegetable assortment is not as wide as yours. But it does seem to be working. I do let the kids have special treats-like when they are going to birthday parties and Hot Dog Day at school — but they have cut down the portions. Again thank you for all your help.

LOW-CARB
PRODUCTS AND
SUPPORT NETWORKS

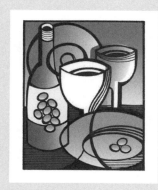

Low-Carb Products and Support Networks

The manufacture of low-carb products in the food and supplement industry has contributed to a dramatic increase in the variety of low-carb products currently available. When we first started eating slow-carb foods we could find low-carb products only in health food and natural food stores. Today we find many of these products on the shelves of our neighborhood grocery store. We have tested many of the new products for taste, value, and availability in both the Canadian and U.S. markets, specialty stores, and on-line. We list below many of the Web addresses of these new resources as well as the Web addresses of support groups.

Though these products are convenient, we caution readers to be careful and to read the labels closely as the products may have higher carb content than is obvious at a casual glance. You have to be especially careful to take into account the serving size for which the carb content is listed. Low-carb pizza, muffins, and cookies can have substantially more carbs than reported on the labels. Unfortunately the U.S. FDA doesn't yet have standards for low-carb labeling and there is no monitoring system in place, which leaves consumers vulnerable to inaccurate information. Use these products sparingly and with caution. Eating fresh products and foods that are cooked at home gives us the security of knowing exactly what we are getting.

Most low-carb products are marketed and sold using the net carb content of the product, a method that subtracts the fiber in the foods from the total carbs to determine the net carb. Manufacturers also deduct the carb content of glycerine and sugar alcohols (which can promote a laxative effect) that most of us don't absorb. However, many people do not tolerate products made with these ingredients and may experience a weight loss plateau or even a gain in weight as a result. These products may also stimulate food cravings, especially the sweet low-carb products like ice cream, cookies, and chocolates. Although we have tried many of these products, and some we keep on hand for special occasions, in general we prefer to eat and prepare fresh foods so that we can be 100 percent sure of the ingredients and our ability to digest the foods without any unwanted side effects. We are cognizant of the fact that manufacturers are improving low-carb products daily. Concerns today may well be dispelled next week. Your best defence is to read labels and keep yourself informed. For these reasons we caution you to experiment slowly with these products and ask questions.

We have noted concerns and comments on taste and side effects based on personal experience. Taste is subjective; you may like some products we didn't enjoy. There are so many new products on the market we have had to limit our reviews to the most popular. If you want to know more, visit the manufacturers' Web sites, or the sites for specialty stores and support groups.

Protein Powders

These protein powders mix with either milk or water to make a protein shake for a quick and easy breakfast, lunch replacement, or snack. Mix two scoops of powder with two tablespoons of heavy or light cream and fill the rest of the container (either a glass or a blender attachment) with water. This adds only one gram of carb to your total carb count. A full glass of milk can add anywhere from 10 to 14 grams of carb depending on the producer and type of milk you choose. Choose a protein powder with no more than two to three grams of carbohydrate per serving. Brands that blend simply with a shake of the container are easier and more portable than those that require a blender. A teaspoon of peppermint or almond extract enhances the flavor.

To Diet For is a Canadian brand of protein powder that comes in vanilla, strawberry, and chocolate flavors. It is now available in our neighborhood grocery store, and on shelves in health food stores and drugstores. It is not widely available in the U.S. See the company Web site at www.nulifevitamins.com.

Designer Protein comes in vanilla, strawberry, and chocolate flavors, but requires a blender or immersion blender to get properly mixed, so there are no lumps (ugh!) in the shake.

Precision IsoPro is another low-carb protein shake that mixes well in a glass with lid. We have found it in the GNC (General Nutrition Centers) in both Canada and the U.S. (sold as IsoPure in the U.S.). This brand is the most economical of all the protein shakes we have tried and comes in vanilla, chocolate, and strawberry. It is very low in carbs, with only 1.4 grams per serving. The GNC stores also have a low-carb whey protein mix that is economical and can be used in muffin recipes.

Trader Joe's (in the United States) have a store brand protein powder that has no carbohydrates at all, according to the label. It is a very inexpensive powder and has no flavor enhancements. This makes it a slightly unpleasant shake to drink, unless you add a little unsweetened cocoa, some Splenda, or a few fresh strawberries to provide some extra flavor. It also requires a blender to get properly mixed.

Dr. Atkins has produced a premixed shake that comes in individual containers, and also a protein powder available in grocery stores. As with other premixed shakes, the cost of a single serving is considerably higher than with the shakes that you mix yourself.

Protein Bars

This product line has expanded dramatically over the past couple of years. Protein bars are small, relatively inexpensive, portable, and make great slow-carb meal replacements or snacks. ConsumerLab.com, an independent evaluator of nutrition products and dietary supplements in White Plains, New York, announced in October 2001 that "60 percent of nutrition bars fail to meet claims." They say that of the 30 protein bars, low-carb bars, and other similar products they tested, only 12 accurately lived up to the claims made on their labels with respect to calories, fat, carbohydrates, sugars, proteins, cholesterol, and sodium. Further, 50 percent, or 15 of the 30 products they tested, exceeded the levels of carbohydrate on the label by as much as 20 grams. This miscalculation was found in the testing to have occurred even among those bars that were labeled low-carb.

Simultaneously, the U.S. FDA ruled that glycerine is a carbohydrate and must be reported as such. Prior to this ruling, many of the manufacturers of these products did not include glycerine or the sugar alcohols in their carbohydrate content. The FDA ruling led to a marketing ploy to promote the net grams of carb rather than the total carbs. Use them sparingly, particularly at the beginning of your weight loss plan. The recipe in this book for homemade low-carb bars has between four to six net grams of carbohydrate in a single serving. It is higher than the commercial products, but you can be confident of every ingredient in the bars, and therefore the carb content. The homemade low-carb bars are also considerably less expensive than the commercial ones.

Atkins Advantage Bars are found in grocery stores and health food stores everywhere. The Advantage bar claims to have 2 grams net carbohydrate per bar and uses Splenda as the main sweetener, rather than aspartame. These bars come in many flavors, including Almond Brownie. Dr. Atkins has a Web site at www.atkins.ca.

Ultimate Lo Carb Bar and Strive are manufactured by Biochem and claim to have only two or three grams of net carbohydrate respectively. They come in a variety of flavors, including Chocolate Nut Brownie. However, the bars vary dramatically in texture (from smooth and creamy to dry as dust) and flavor (from very rich chocolate to bland), depending on the batch. The product has also become difficult to purchase in Canada. The Strive Crunchy Chocolate Smores bars are very good. Their Web site is www.biochemfitness.com.

Carb Solutions is a popular newcomer on the low-carb market and available widely in health food and grocery stores. There are many flavors and they advertise a net carb content of only two grams. These bars have a chocolate-like coating that make them impractical for carrying in warm weather. Further information is available at www.CarbSolutions.com.

To Diet For is made by the same Canadian company that makes the protein shake, and their bars taste very good. The company does reduce the carb content by the amount of glycerine in the bars, but the carb content is still 15 grams per serving, which is a little high. Information about these products can be found on the company Web site at www.nulifevitamins.com.

Doctor's CarbRite Diet is a line of protein bars that claim 2.5 grams of net carb per serving and maintain they use no hydrogenated oils and no artificial sweeteners, but these bars do contain sugar alcohols. There are many different flavors, including Chocolate Mint Cookie, which tastes like a chocolate bar. The Web site is www.UniversalNutrition.com.

Think Thin Low-Carb Diet Bars advertise only three grams of net carb per serving and are marketed to the diabetic community as well as the low-carb community. The company that distributes this product is Prime Health with a Web site at www.thinkproducts.com.

3 Carb Protein Bar is manufactured by BioX and distributed in Canada by Nutrition Zone Products Inc., which has a Web site at www.nutritionzone.com. The product comes in many flavors and contains both glycerine and sugar alcohols in various quantities, which affect the taste. These bars are readily available in health food and grocery stores.

EAS AdvantEdge CarbControl Nutrition is a new bar made by EAS in Golden, Colorado. The label lists four grams of impact carbs in each bar. The flavors include Apple Cinnamon (good!), Chocolate Peanut Butter, Chocolate Chip Brownie, and Blueberry. We wonder about the real carb content, and these bars can be difficult to find. The Web site is www.eas.com.

Precision is manufactured by Sci Fit and advertises itself as the premiere low-carb bar with only two grams of net carb. These bars are produced in Canada but we were unable to find a Web site.

Designer Whey Protein has a Creamy Peanut Butter Chocolate bar that is quite tasty. These protein bars are manufactured by Next Proteins in Carlsbad, California.

Pria Carb Select are new in 2004 and are manufactured by the same company that makes Power Bars. They are currently available in Peanut Butter Caramel Nut, Caramel Nut Brownie, and Cookies and Cream. They taste like a chocolate bar and report only 2 grams of impact carbs (the same thing as net carbs) per bar. They are stocked by Costco and sold by the carton, which makes them the most economical on the market. Their Web site is www.powerbar.com.

The following sample is a representative overview of some typical products on the market, though many are simply too expensive to be worth the cost (a single low-carb chocolate chip cookie for $5.00 U.S.!). Most of these products are made with the same glycerine and sugar alcohols that are in the low-carb protein bars. Please experiment slowly when you are introducing these products into your meal plan to make sure you tolerate them without side effect.

Cereals and Granola

Keto Crisp (vanilla) and **Keto Cocoa Crisp** (chocolate) have only 3 grams of carb per serving and do not contain any aspartame, saccharin, or sugar. This cereal is made with all natural products and has a very pleasant taste. Slice two or three strawberries on top and serve with a little light cream or whole milk. These products contain 22 grams of soy protein in a serving. We tried a nut and oat flake cereal made by the Keto Food company, but it was very dry in texture and had a funny aftertaste. The company also makes a low-carb powdered skim milk substitute for cooking and has more than 100 low-carb products found in health food stores or on their Web site at www.ketofoods.com.

Wild Cherry Nutrageous granola has two grams of effective carb per serving though it is made with the sugar alcohols.

LowCarb Success has a number of products, including Flax O Meal hot cereals, and a Web site at www.lowcarbsuccess.org. Flax O Meal instant hot cereals are tasty and very easy to make; they come in a variety of flavors, including Vanilla Almond and Strawberry. They are very high in fiber and protein, contain no sugar alcohols, and have a net carb content of just 2 grams of carb per serving.

Breads, Wraps, and Baking Mixes

Increasing numbers of low-carb breads and wraps are found in the health food and specialty stores, some with as low as three grams of net carbs per slice. More and more bakeries are producing low-carb breads and many stores keep sugar-free bread for their diabetic customers. Be sure to check the label and nutrition information before trying these new breads. We caution you to start with these products slowly, to see how your body reacts to them.

Tumaro's LowinCarb Gourmet Tortilla are very dry and cannot be folded without ripping.

CarbOLé Tortillas taste quite good and are soft and pliable.

"Atkins Approved" Wrap at Subway is quite tasty. The nutrition information suggests that the wrap on its own has only five grams of net carb. The total net carb of your wrap will vary depending on the vegetables and other ingredients that you request.

Baking mixes for low-carb bread, muffins, and cakes tend to be expensive, often don't taste very good, and sometimes boast inaccurate labeling of carb content. Recently some large low-carb manufacturers like CarbSense have begun offering mixes for biscuits, pie crust, corn muffins, cookies, pancakes, and pizza crust. Although this is an improvement over what has been available, homemade is still best in our opinion.

Chocolate

Most low-carb chocolate treats are made with the sugar alcohols, so less is more.

Pure DeLite chocolate bars come in a wide variety of flavors, including milk chocolate and dark chocolate. They are made from Belgian chocolate and are sugar and lactose free. Each bar contains only 1.1 grams of carb. The company also makes a low-carb chewy chocolate and licorice bar with three net grams of carb. The bars are a good size for a single serving, are reasonably priced, and are found in health food and drugstores everywhere. The Web address is www.puredeliteproducts.com.

Ross chocolate bars, manufactured in British Columbia, are made with Belgian chocolate and have no sugar added. They come in Raspberry Delight, Crunchy Delight, and White Chocolate among others. These bars have no sugar added and contain 2.7 grams of carbohydrate per bar, though information is not available on the label. They are a good size, reasonably priced, and found in health food and drugstores throughout Canada. They have a distributor in the U.S. with a Web site at www.lowcarbchocolate.com. Ross Chocolates are identified on several Web sites though they do not have their own.

Endulge products are made for the Atkins company, but we find them more expensive than other varieties. They are promoted as having only two grams net carb per serving and make peanut butter cups and caramel nut chews as well. All Atkins products can be found at www.atkinscenter.com.

Carbolite Foods were one of the first to make low-carb chocolates. They have two grams of net carb per serving with fairly high concentrations of sugar alcohols. They come in a variety of flavors, including milk chocolate, chocolate crisp, and chocolate peanut butter. These bars are reasonably priced and widely available in 7-Eleven stores as well as grocery and drugstores. Their Web site is www.carbolitedirect.com.

Specialty chocolates are now frequently available in a sugar-free form. They taste great, but the carb content varies widely.

Rocky Mountain Chocolate Factory sugar-free chocolates averaged 15 grams of carbohydrate per chocolate!

Purdy's sugar-free chocolate truffles have only four grams of carb per chocolate and are made for the diabetic community — delicious!

Russell Stover sells fancy sugar-free chocolates with full nutrition information on the boxes. They announced a full line of low-carb chocolates in the summer of 2004.

Ice Cream

Breyers Low-Carb Ice Cream is creamy, tastes great, and a half-cup serving has about four grams of net carb. Breyers is sweetened with Splenda. It comes in vanilla, chocolate, and strawberry. In Canada the product is called Breyers Smart Scoop Carb Zone and it is in a bright orange/yellow rectangular container. In the U.S. the product is Breyers Carb Smart and the container is blue. We do not recommend eating it during the weight loss period lest it stimulate food cravings, cause a stall in your weight loss, or have a laxative effect.

Klondike makes tasty frozen low-carb ice cream bars found in several grocery stores. The fudge bars have three grams net carb per bar and come six to a box.

The ice cream bars have five grams net carb per bar and also come six to a box.

Dairy Queen has low-sugar frozen products that they manufacture primarily for diabetics, but they are higher in carbs than other products, averaging about 17 grams per serving. They contain both sorbitol, a sugar alcohol, and aspartame.

Fruit Drinks

Talking Rain Diet Ice Botanicals are low-carb drinks made with Splenda that purport to have zero grams of carb. We are a little skeptical about the zero grams because even Splenda has some carb content. They are sold in Costco by the case and each case contains peach, strawberry kiwi, cranberry raspberry, and key lime.

Hansen's Diet Drinks come in peach, kiwi strawberry, and ginger ale and are available in many outlets in the U.S., but we haven't seen them in Canada yet. They use Splenda as a sweetener.

Diet Snapple iced tea and other fruitlike drinks come in many flavors and have very low carb content.

Health food stores and the diabetic aisles in your neighborhood grocery are great places to find new products. Some of these products may be introduced into the marketplace in the U.S. before they are available in Canada, so if they aren't north of the border already it should be only a matter of time. Grocery chains keep track of the number of requests for certain products so let them know what you'd like them to stock.

Helpful Websites

Several generic low-carb sites provide a wide range of services such as forums and product and research information. These sites change addresses, Web masters, topics of interest quickly, but at the time of our publication all of these sites were working and dedicated to low-carb topics.

www.slowcarbforlife.com is our own Web site that provides regular research and product updates as well as newly developed slow-carb recipes and readers' questions and answers.

www.lowcarb.ca based in Ottawa is one of the best administered and easiest sites to navigate. There is no charge to join. The discussions about product and research information and member forums get thousands of hits from all over North America, England, New Zealand, and Australia every month. The Web master sends out regular reviews to all registered users to highlight active topics (threads). It is a very supportive environment where lay people share their personal experience.

www.geocities.com/alabastercat/lowcarb.html is the ultimate low-carb resource page. It is a large, well-organized collection of low-carb links.

www.atkinscenter.com is the general Atkins Web site that discusses the Atkins diet and products; it provides a lot of low-carb information.

www.lowcarbcentre.com is both an online store and a network of stores complete with delis, located in British Columbia and Ontario, with new stores opening all the time. Check their Web site for the latest locations and products.

www.carbsmart.com is an on-line store based in California. It has a wide selection of products.

www.netrition.com is a general nutrition on-line store that is not low-carb specific, but does include many low-carb products. The site has great information on nutrition and current research.

www.diabeticdepot.com in Calgary, Alberta, has a wonderful selection of everyday items dedicated to slow-carb living. You can purchase items either in the store or on-line.

www.musclememory.ca is a full-service food store with low-carb products called Low-Carb Solutions in Tsawwassen, British Columbia.

www.nal.usda.gov/fnic/foodcomp/search/ allows you to search the USDA Nutrient Database for Standard Reference, the ultimate database of nutritional contents of food.

www.fitday.com allows you to record your daily food intake, should you wish to do this on-line, rather than in your Food Diary.

www.lono.us was designed to allow user entry of their own recipes. LoNo then cross-references each ingredient against the entire USDA Food Ingredient Database of over 6600 items. The result is a neatly formatted recipe with ingredients, directions, and calorie, carbohydrate, fat, fiber, sodium, calcium, potassium, iron, protein, and cholesterol nutrient values by portion and for the entire recipe.

A recent edition of *LowCarb Living* announced Total Carb Count Certified, in which independent labs test low-carb products from various manufacturers and provide a certification seal of approval if the carb content shows the labeling to be accurate and honest. We hope this attempt to standardize the testing and labeling of low-carb products is accepted by manufacturers and consumers. See www.lclmag.com for more information.

- -

Karen and David: Thunder Bay, Ontario
October 31, 2002

Dear Harv and Patricia:
My husband and I are two of the converted. We have inspired four of our friends to adopt your way of eating. My husband was told by his doctor to lose weight or be taken out on a flatbed truck. I am proud to say he has met his target weight. I have lost 26 pounds with a bit more to go. My husband's cardiologist is thrilled with him and asked all kinds of questions about your book. My husband gave him the title and your Web site. His doctor said he'll use my husband as his poster boy for how to lose weight sensibly. Had to let you hear our success.

May 28, 2003
Greetings from Thunder Bay with an update on our progress. All is well — our goals have been met and maintained. We have introduced several friends to your eating program and they all have had success. We are most proud of my sister and brother-in-law who just started. Each has lost over 20 pounds. They both have chronic health concerns and are feeling so much better on your program.

David has been asked by his cardiologist to attend a dinner at a weekend retreat they have for all their cardiac patients. They want him to tell other patients how he has lost his weight and kept it off. He'll be talking about your books and will give out your Web site. Even if only a few adopt your program he'll feel successful. Bye for now.

REFERENCES
AND ANNOTATED
BIBLIOGRAPHY

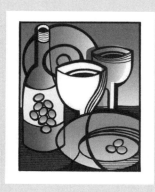

References and Annotated Bibliography

This chapter is devoted to providing a shorthand review of 18 of the popular diet books on the market today and a list of journal entries quoted in the text for your reference. Even though each diet takes a slightly different approach as interpreted by the author, the scientific basis remains the same for all. It is not our intention to convince you that one diet is better than the other, although we express our own opinion about the merits of various approaches.

Agatston, Arthur, M.D. *The South Beach Diet*. New York: Random House, 2003.
We had barely gotten into the first chapter of this book when we found ourselves checking the publication date: 2003. The principles in this book are so similar to those we set forth in our first book, *Easy Low-Carb Living*, published in 2002, we found our ideas echoed in the first five lines, "*The South Beach Diet* is not low-carb. Nor is it low fat. *The South Beach Diet* teaches you to rely on the right carbs and the right fats — the good ones —and enables you to live quite happily without the bad carbs and bad fats." Dr. Agatston writes the book from his perspective as a cardiologist with the objective of preventing heart attacks and strokes, despite its popularity with those trying to lose weight to improve their appearance. Dr. Agatston's disillusionment with the American Heart Association's low-fat, high-carb diet and its lack of success convinced him that you can "save your life" by removing the bad carbohydrates from your diet. He found people trying to follow the Atkins diet were put off by having to give up fruits and vegetables (our experience as well) and he didn't feel it necessary to eat all the saturated fats recommended by Atkins to be successful.

Dr. Agatston offers two simple strategies to stop ourselves from overeating: "We can eat the foods (and combinations of foods) that cause gradual rather than sharp increases and decreases in blood sugar and we can learn to anticipate hypoglycemia and avert it with the timely consumption of snacks. This one is crucial: It takes much less food to prevent hypoglycemia than it does to resolve it." He goes on to describe "central obesity" as "excess weight concentrated mainly in a rounded, protruding waistline. Often on individuals with the face, arms, and legs you'd expect to find on someone thinner." This condition is "a serious warning of unhealthy blood chemistry today and cardiac trouble ahead." Many people with this condition have pre-diabetes, which, according to the National Cholesterol Education Program, is high cholesterol, high ratio of bad cholesterol to good, high blood pressure, central obesity, high triglycerides, and small LDL (bad cholesterol) particles.

In our opinion this is a very good book for anyone interested in following a diet to prevent heart attacks and strokes, and will also serve those whose main objective is weight loss and weight control. However, it offers little practical guidance and leaves readers on their own more than most might like. This weakness is somewhat overcome by its detailed meal planning and 122 recipes.

Atkins, Robert C., M.D. *Atkins for Life*. New York: St. Martin's, 2003.
What a difference three or four years can make. The difference between this book (published in 2003) and his previous version (published in 1999) is quite remarkable. This book presents the Dr. Atkins diet in significantly modified terms. He appears less defensive about his approach, no longer justifying his point of view to mainstream doctors and nutritionists. He now acknowledges that not everyone needs to reduce his or her carb intake to the 20 grams of carb per day level to succeed in weight loss. He has introduced the concept of controlled carbs versus low-carb (p. 21). Instead of advising the reader to eat as much protein and fat, as he or she needs to satisfy hunger, he now gives guidance as to portion control (p. 76). Surprisingly, he also recommends less protein (p. 158) than he did previously and suggests the type of protein to select to ensure adequate intake of all the essential amino acids. He has not recommended any decrease in saturated fat intake. A new nomenclature called ACE (Atkins Carbohydrate Equilibrium) is introduced to identify the level of carb intake an individual can consume each day without gaining or losing weight. Another new term called AGR (Atkins Glycemic Rating) is presented to eliminate the need for readers to sort through the effect of Glycemic Index (GI) and Glycemic Load (GL) for different foods.

In our view this book is much more user-friendly than *Dr. Atkins' New Diet Revolution*. It is easier to read, more attractively laid out, and presents information that will be helpful to readers. As with most other books on this subject, however, the reader doesn't get the advice and guidance that comes from an author who knows from personal experience what works and what doesn't.

Atkins, Robert C., M.D. *Dr. Atkins' New Diet Revolution*. New York: HarperCollins, 1999.

This is another one of several books that Dr. Atkins has in print. He is undoubtedly the best known and most published of all proponents of the low-carb approach to diet. His work and opinions have come under much criticism over the years, but as research catches up it appears that Dr. Atkins may have been ahead of his time.

The basis of Dr. Atkins's plan is that dramatic restriction of carbohydrate intake will cause the body to enter a condition he calls Benign Dietary Ketosis (BDK). In order to get into BDK it is necessary to reduce carbohydrates to below 40 grams per day. This is difficult, given that most people in our North American society consume somewhere in the order of 300 grams per day. Being in ketosis simply means that your body is burning your fat stores as a source of fuel. Reduced availability of sugar (sucrose) due to decreased carbohydrate intake forces the body into ketosis.

The appetite suppression that accompanies carbohydrate reduction coupled with the higher proportion of fat in the diet provides increased satiation and makes it easier to lose weight. That said, there are three aspects of Dr. Atkins' program about which you should be concerned. First, he advocates a weight loss program that begins with less than 20 grams of carbohydrate a day. We believe that most people can achieve successful weight loss at 30 to 45 grams. Second, his advice for vitamin supplementation is extremely complex and difficult to follow without medical help. Third, he promotes his own product line. You can also follow an effective and healthy low-carb lifestyle with foods readily available in your local market. This is an important book for anyone interested in knowing the low-carb mechanism from the guru himself.

Brand-Miller, Jennie, Johanna Burani, Kaye Foster-Powell, and Susanna Holt. *The New Glucose Revolution: Complete Guide to Glycemic Index (GI) Values.* **New York: Marlowe & Company, 2003.**

This is a small companion book to the popular *The New Glucose Revolution* and will be most useful for people with diabetes, heart disease, Syndrome X, and obesity. It is also a helpful quick reference for anyone wanting to put the Glycemic Index (GI) into practice. It presents an A to Z list of individual foods for easy reference, a comprehensive list of foods and food categories for more in-depth knowledge, and a simple food-category list in order of low to high GI value for quick comparisons. The authors advise that you can use the different tables to find the GI value of your favorite food, to compare foods within the same category (for instance, two types of bread) to see which food has a lower GI value, to improve your diet by finding low GI substitutes for high GI foods, to find the lowest GI value within a food group, to compare the GI values of food groups, to put together a low GI meal, to shop for low GI foods, and to check the GI values of products. If you are prepared to invest some time in becoming quite knowledgeable about the Glycemic Index (GI) this is a good resource, but it cannot be read like a Carb Counter or a cookbook.

D'Adamo, Dr. Peter J. *Live Right For Your Type.* **New York: G.P. Putnam's Sons, 2001.**

This is a fascinating book, but much too complicated for the average person seeking guidance about healthy eating for weight loss and maintenance. For those who are interested in a detailed set of guidelines or those who are struggling with chronic illness, Dr. D'Adamo's book will be more useful. His basic thesis is that our blood type (O, A, B, or AB) and whether we are what he calls "secretors" or "non-secretors" determine our personality, our response to stress, our emotional stability, how we digest our food, our metabolism, our immunity, and our toxicity. For those who are Blood Type O or B he recommends a lifestyle similar to the slow-carb program we offer. Those who are Blood Type A or AB will require more soy and fish for protein sources and significantly less chicken or red meat. This is the second book regarding diet and blood type by this author. Anyone who is interested in learning more about this approach will want to read both books.

Diamond, Harvey and Marilyn. *Fit For Life*. New York: Warner Books, 1987.

This book promotes food combining as a weight control mechanism, a more scientific approach than the one taken by Suzanne Somers. Harvey Diamond studied natural hygiene for over 10 years, receiving a doctorate in nutritional science from the American College of Health Science in Austin, Texas. He outlines three natural body cycles and suggests ways to eat that will enhance the body's ability to deal with each: "on a daily basis we take in food (appropriation), we absorb and use some of that food (assimilation), and we get rid of what we don't use (elimination)" (p. 26). He asserts that appropriation (eating and digesting) occurs from noon to 8 p.m., assimilation from 8 p.m. to 4 a.m., and elimination from 4 a.m. to noon (p. 27).

This method suggests that you eat nothing but fresh fruit and fruit juices until noon — ever! As with Somers' method of food combining, the authors suggest you never eat fruit except on its own because it passes very quickly through the stomach and into the intestines where it is easily absorbed by the body. Because fruit has such a high water content, it requires less energy than other foods to be digested. You must wait after eating other foods before you are allowed to eat fruit (timetables provided).

Both authors are vegetarian and advocate this choice in addition to eating most vegetables raw, rather than cooked or processed in any way, in order to get the most nutrients. They also present a formula or ladder of foods to be consumed in order to maximize energy. At the bottom of the ladder are fruits and fruit juices, then fresh vegetable salads and juices (lunch), then steamed vegetables with raw nuts and seeds, then grains, breads, potatoes, and legumes, and finally meat, chicken, fish, and dairy. They claim that the highest energy levels will be achieved on days that only fruits and vegetables are consumed.

Marilyn Diamond is a nutritionist who has developed a number of recipes to complement this approach, including a four-week menu plan to get you started. It is not suggested as a short-term solution to either health problems or weight control.

In general we remain unconvinced and find the idea of eating only fruit until noon to be too difficult and food combining too complicated. However, anyone interested in the theory and practice of food combining will be interested in this book.

Eades, Dr. Michael R. and Dr. Mary Dan. *The Protein Power Lifeplan*. New York: Warner Books, 2000.

This is a low-carbohydrate, high-protein diet plan for weight loss, rather than a low-fat approach. The authors explain that, "Clearly the low fat diet hasn't been the panacea that many had hoped for; in fact, it has turned out to be a dismal failure, a fact admitted publicly in 1996 by most of the world's experts in nutritional research" (p. xix). The authors suggest that carbohydrates are virtually the only foods that cause people to binge because carbohydrates activate a reward center in our brains that overrides common sense and feelings of being full. They review the results of any diet high in carbohydrates, and there is an extensive section on various medical conditions and their improvement with reduced carbohydrate consumption. There is also considerable discussion of the insulin mechanism and hyperinsulinemia, how cholesterol impacts our health, antioxidants and their use, and how diet impacts the autoimmune system.

The authors have developed a formula to demonstrate that the carbohydrate left over after we take out the fiber, the Effective Carbohydrate Content (ECC), is "Total Carbohydrate - Dietary Fiber = Effective Carbohydrate" (p. 323). To use this formula in calculating your daily carbohydrate allowance, you will of course need to know the dietary fiber content of the carbohydrates. The authors list low-carbohydrate vegetables and fruits and provide some guidance with respect to the fiber content and its impact on daily consumption.

They also suggest that we can get all the nutrients we need without eating any grains or potatoes because many of the nutrients we need are fat-soluble and only need small amounts of fat to absorb them. They suggest that many of the cancer-fighting nutrients, such as antioxidants, cannot be well absorbed by the body unless they are eaten with small amounts of fat. They recommend that green salad always be eaten with a dressing made of extra virgin olive oil, or canola oil, to ensure the absorption of these nutrients. They also recommend that we drizzle olive oil or butter on steamed vegetables.

They hypothesize that our stomachs and digestive tract were not designed to deal with grains and grain products, and that our ancestors were healthier because they ate only meat, vegetables, fruits, and nuts. The authors review issues related to fructose, the simple sugar found in fruit, and its absorption into the blood stream, and talk about the proliferation of products on the market that use fructose as the sweetening agent. While the quantities of fructose found in honey and fruits are relatively small, the amount added to commercially prepared foods is considerable. They blame the rise of diabetes and obesity in North America on this fact.

This is a very popular low-carb diet and we know many have followed its recommendations with considerable success, but it is difficult to read and to implement their plan effectively. Furthermore, although there is a lot of good information in this book, we disagree with some of its recommendations. For example, the authors caution against the use of sunblock and instead suggest we spend time building up a tolerance to the sun to facilitate the production of vitamin D and melanin. This recommendation is in direct conflict with our knowledge of the damaging effects of the sun and the risk of skin cancer.

Gallop, Rick. *The GI (Glycemic Index) Diet*. Toronto: Random House Canada, 2002.

This is a low-carb diet book written by a layperson based on his personal journey. The author organizes carbohydrate foods according to their Glycemic Index (GI). Those with a high GI are coded red to be avoided. Those with a mid-range GI are placed in the yellow group and are to be used with caution during maintenance, not during weight loss. The low GI carbohydrates are classified green, meaning go ahead. This is meant to make it easy for readers to know what they can eat and what is off limits. However, because the reader isn't personally involved in developing the list he or she is less likely to really understand it.

Gallop focuses on the importance of calories, sticking close to the traditional wisdom that calories in equal calories out. We disagree. He recommends several times that readers use aspartame for sweetener. We think this is bad advice. The author tells his readers to make carbohydrates 55 percent of their calories (p. 25). In our view that is too high. We think the focus should be on the grams of carb, not the percentage of calories. Gallop writes from a low-fat perspective, giving advice like "avoid cheeses like the plague," and make sure to use "low fat" salad dressings. This short book is easy to read and ideal for someone who wants to follow rules and trust that somebody else has done all the work. It will not suit the individual who wants to understand why they gain or lose weight.

Haas, Elson M., MD. *The False Fat Diet*. New York: Ballantine Books, 2001.

This is a book based on the premise that extra fat, especially around the middle of the body, is "false fat" as a result of an allergic reaction to various foods. Our metabolisms affect our ability to digest certain foods, so Dr. Haas treats patients for obesity and other physical ailments by determining their food sensitivities and eliminating the foods that cause reactions. He maintains our food reactions (p. 50):

- cause fluid to surround invading food particles
- release hormones that cause fluid retention
- make intestinal membranes swell
- disrupt cell chemistry, causing fluid storage
- cause capillaries to leak fluids
- cause gas production.

Consuming foods we react to causes the immune system to work overtime; if we eliminate these reactive foods from our diet, the immune system is strengthened and better able to cope with other complaints. If you suffer from hay fever and are regularly eating foods you are sensitive to, you may unwittingly be exacerbating your symptoms. If you eliminate the reactive foods from your diet the hay fever might disappear because your immune system is freed up to cope more effectively with pollens in the air.

The author lists seven foods that are most often the cause of reactions: dairy products, wheat, sugar, soy, peanuts, corn, and eggs. He recommends an elimination diet to help you determine if you react to any of these foods, and a series of increasingly restrictive diets will determine your level of reaction. By reintroducing the seven sensitive foods, one at a time, you isolate your body's response. Many of the processed foods we consume today are full of chemicals, additives, fillers, and high quantities of these seven foods. He recommends we eat unprocessed whole foods such as fresh fruit and vegetables, fish, poultry, nuts, and rice. The book provides a food reaction reference guide and some interesting recipes. The author explains that food reactions can create metabolic roadblocks to weight loss by "Slowing the metabolic rate, increasing the hormones that cause weight gain, creating hypoglycemia, depressing energy, and contributing to illness" (p. 63).

This is a program that recognizes the failure of the low-fat approach to diets. "Ironically, many people who have tried hard to eat wisely have become hypoglycemic, because they are eating too many carbohydrates and not enough protein. People who live on carbohydrates that include mostly fruits, grains, and starchy vegetables become hypoglycemic more easily than people who have a more balanced diet, with higher amounts of protein" (p. 65). Dr. Haas says that of all the food cravings, "carbohydrate craving is the most common" (p. 61). Anyone who thinks they may have food sensitivities will want to read this volume.

Heavin, Gary. *Curves.* New York: G.P. Putnam's Sons, 2003.

We were pleasantly surprised in Chapter 7, Nutrition for a Great Body (pp. 130–146), to discover Heavin discussing good fat, bad fat, trans fat, slow carbs, and fiber. Heavin's background as a fitness instructor reinforces that one pound of muscle burns 50 calories per day at rest. He says that most North Americans lose five to 10 pounds of muscle per decade as a result of inactivity (p. 10). Losing weight through calorie reduction results in as much as one third of the weight loss being muscle rather than fat so muscle bulk is an important component of effective weight management. Heavin's premise is that long-term weight management is achieved by controlling the body's metabolic rate in part by muscle bulk and fitness and in part by controlling caloric intake. He suggests that if an individual's weight loss plateaus, he or she should eat more calories, not less, to convince the body it does not need to preserve body fat because it has interpreted the calorie loss as starvation.

Adjusting the metabolic rate in this way is the basis of the long-term maintenance (Phase III) of the Curves weight loss program. The author advises that daily weigh-ins are necessary to identify when weight has increased by three to five pounds. If this happens on a diet of 2500 calories per day, it is necessary to go back on the weight loss program (Phase I). Return to normal eating is acceptable as soon as the ideal weight is again attained. The author suggests that an individual can maintain his or her ideal weight by eating normally except for one or two days of dieting per month.

The focus of this book is exclusively on weight without adequate focus on a healthy eating pattern. Many readers are apt to be seduced by dieting two or three days a month, but they would be better served by a permanent lifestyle change that provides long-term weight maintenance. We also don't agree with the proposition of daily weigh-in. If the reader can avoid taking the easy road and focusing on only weight, there is other good information here.

Heller, Dr. Rachael F., and Dr. Richard F. *The Carbohydrate Addict's Diet*. New York: Penguin Books, 1993.

This popular diet book suggests that each of us is addicted to carbohydrates to some degree. The authors have developed a test to determine whether an individual has: 1) Doubtful Addiction; 2) Mild Carbohydrate Addiction; 3) Moderate Carbohydrate Addiction; or 4) Severe Carbohydrate Addiction. If you test positive for addiction they suggest you follow their diet.

Two factors are at play: how many times a day carbohydrates are consumed and how much time is spent consuming them. The Hellers claim that if addicts consume their daily carbohydrate load at one sitting (called a Reward Meal) in less than an hour, they will avoid hyperinsulinism. They don't suggest reducing the amount of carbohydrate consumed at that one sitting, but the other meals in the day should be high in fiber and fat and low in carbs.

We recommend that the total daily carbohydrate intake be kept low overall rather than splurged or disregarded at the Reward Meal. The test for carbohydrate addiction is worth taking but we have serious reservations about the Reward Meals. Anyone who feels that they may be addicted to carbohydrates should read this book.

Kenton, Leslie. *The X Factor Diet*. London: Random House, 2002.

The author of this book is a journalist who explains difficult concepts much better than most scientists. She tracks the historical changes (agricultural revolution) in eating patterns to convince us of the importance of a return to low-carb eating. The name of her book refers to Syndrome X, a series of conditions associated with insulin resistance. She has developed a diet program with two components, Ketogenics and Insulin Balance. Ketogenics is a diet designed for those individuals who are significantly overweight (fat constitutes more than 35 percent of body mass in females, and more than 22 percent in males). She suggests that the Ketogenic program will significantly decrease the fat level, overcome insulin resistance, increase metabolic rate, decrease sugar cravings, eliminate constant hunger, detoxify the body, and increase energy levels.

The Insulin Balance program is designed for those who are normal weight to moderately overweight. She claims that this program will decrease fat levels, stave off aging, increase lean body mass to fat ratio, detoxify the body, and increase energy levels. The main differences between the two programs are that the Ketogenic program places greater emphasis on foods that have carbohydrates with a low Glycemic Index (GI), has more protein, and includes Omega3 fatty acids. The author encourages the consumption of micro-filtered whey protein concentrates or whey peptide blends, since other products will not have retained the essential molecular structure necessary to be effective in the body.

Kenton's diets are not simple, but her 27-page chapter "X Factor Diet Idiots' Guide" helps. We have no doubt the diet will work, but those who choose to follow it need to be serious students.

McGraw, Dr. Phil. *The Ultimate Weight Solution: The 7 Keys to Weight Loss Freedom.* New York: The Free Press, 2003.

As one would expect, Dr. Phil approaches this subject from a psychological perspective. Dr. Phil's 7 Keys are:

- Right Thinking unlocks the door to self-control, which "enables you to discard all the toxic messages, replace them with realistic, positive thoughts, then act on the new, more constructive way of engaging the world."
- Healing Feelings unlock the door to emotional control so you can "learn how to break the cycle of overeating in response to emotions and stress. You can't eliminate emotional triggers and stress — they're facts of life — but you can learn how to heal counterproductive responses to life's challenges and gain a new sense of control over your eating."
- A No Fail Environment gives you external control "to shape, design, and manage your environment so that it is virtually impossible for you to fail at weight control."

- Mastery over Food and Impulse Eating will allow you to master habit control so you can "learn how to control and reshape your behavior, first by identifying why you persist in these bad habits, and second, by replacing them with actions designed to weaken their hold over you."
- High-Response Cost, High-Yield Nutrition gives you food control, "an approach to nutritional balance that is nothing short of revolutionary, and amazingly powerful in its simplicity."
- Intentional Exercise provides body control the result of which is "the power to keep pounds at bay with a maximum results workout strategy that you can start slowly and continue at your own pace."
- Your Circle of Support unlocks the door to social control with which "you assemble a support circle of people who will encourage you and provide the accountability you need to achieve your goals."

Dr. Phil cautions that psychologically your "get real" weight has little to do with the numbers on the scale. In his opinion your "get real" weight means: "You like your body and live in it with pride. You are happy and truly at peace with your size. You accept your God-given uniqueness. "You treat your body with respect, care, and love. You like what you see in the mirror every day. You focus your attention on living well, rather than looking good."

We believe there is much more to maintaining a healthy weight than appearance. The health benefits of adopting a slow-carb approach far outweigh the aesthetics. Our biggest disappointment in Dr. Phil's book was that he chose not to embrace low-carb living and opted instead to stick with the traditional mantra of "all things in moderation."

Montignac, Michel. *Eat Yourself Slim*. Quebec: Michel-Ange Publishing, 1999.

This book was published in 1999, before the current popularity of low-carb living, and even then Montignac had it right. Early in the book he says, "we don't gain weight because we eat too much, but because we eat poorly" (p. 19), and spends the first chapter explaining why counting calories is an ineffective way to lose weight. "Reduced calorie weight loss has never been established by science, but we hang onto this myth because the low-calorie diet often produces results at the beginning and it has become big business" (p. 29).

Montignac helps the reader choose good carbs (low GI) instead of bad ones (high GI) and stresses the importance of fiber, which helps the digestive tract to push food through efficiently. Soluble fiber limits digestive absorption, especially of blood lipids. He also offers four possible causes for slow weight loss among women: "stress, which stimulates insulin secretion; hormonal disturbances, especially during adolescence and menopause; thyroid problems, which are rather rare; and excess yoyo dieting" (p. 81).

There are, however, a couple of issues that reflect the fact that the book was written a few years ago. He recommends aspartame as an artificial sweetener rather than Splenda, the newer and safer alternative, and suggests that fruits be eaten separately, a practice that does not have any basis in science. Unfortunately he also fails to recommend eating three snacks every day in addition to three meals. This was surprising since he does make the point that the body will expend more energy digesting food eaten over several meals rather than if it is eaten all at once.

This is an easy book to read at 160 pages and is likely to be enjoyed by anyone looking for another perspective on the GI approach to low-carb eating.

Schwarzbein, Diana, MD. *The Schwarzbein Principle II: The Transition.* **Deerfield Beach, FL: Health Communications, 2002.**
Dr. Schwarzbein is an endocrinologist so she discusses how the hormonal functions of the body determine our overall health and lifespan. She considers the following steps essential to achieving good health:
- Healthy nutrition, including supplementation with vitamins, antioxidants, minerals, and amino and fatty acids, if needed.
- Stress management, including getting enough sleep.
- Tapering off toxic chemicals or avoiding them completely.
- Cross-training exercise.
- Hormone replacement therapy (HRT), if needed.

The author's use of case histories to illustrate her points adds a measure of interest that would otherwise be lacking from this somewhat academic approach.

She also advises that "Contrary to popular belief, you don't get hormones in your food! In order to produce new hormones, you have to eat the right food that has the necessary material for your body to make them. Since hormones are mainly made from proteins, cholesterol, and essential fats, eating a balanced diet is essential for keeping up the production of your hormones" (p. 22). She also makes the important distinction that "the cholesterol in your body that comes from eating cholesterol-rich foods (from red meat for example) and the cholesterol you make in your liver from excess energy (such as refined carbohydrates) are not the same. It is the overproduction of cholesterol in your liver that leads to the type of cholesterol that is easily oxidized (causing damage to your arterial walls) and increases your risk of heart disease" (p. 98).

Most of Dr. Schwarzbein's advice is consistent with what we offer in *Slow Carb for Life*, but she also makes several interesting observations. Since 1993 there has been a dramatic rise in depression caused by malnutrition, especially among women. She attributes this to the low-fat movement and to women trying to stay thin by counting calories. She also cautions that the commonly held belief that a diet too high in protein can contribute to osteoporosis is only half of the story. A diet too low in protein will lack the essential building blocks to form bone, so it will also result in osteoporosis.

This book requires careful reading and study, as it is not easy to keep the complexities of hormonal function clear. It is likely to be most useful for the reader who has embarked on a healthy lifestyle with the guidance of a physician.

Sears, Barry Ph.D. *The Zone.* New York: HarperCollins, 1995.

Sears is a biochemist with a particular interest in diet, biochemistry, and heart disease. He has spent considerable time unraveling the secrets of how the body utilizes food, and what happens at a cellular level when we metabolize food. Although there is some scientific jargon in this book, it is well-written and reasonably easy to understand. The author contends that this diet will enhance physical performance, sharpen mental acuity, and optimize health. He explains, "You must eat food in a controlled fashion and in the proper proportions. The dietary technology required to reach the Zone is as precise as any computer technology. The rules of this dietary technology may appear complicated at first, but

I think once you put them into practice you'll find they're exceptionally easy to follow" (p. 3).

The author provides explanations of the insulin mechanism, the Glycemic Index (GI) of foods, and other mechanisms that contribute to fat storage and disease. There are many interesting anecdotes about athletes with whom the author has tested his approach to diet, but he has also tested it on ordinary individuals and persons suffering from a variety of diseases. Sears contends that following a Zone-favorable diet will have positive effects on heart disease, arthritis, diabetes, blood pressure, and even cancer. (Of course, many of these conditions are equally responsive to a low-carb plan.) The anecdotal evidence is compelling.

This book was not written, nor was this diet developed, primarily for weight loss; weight loss is a side effect. The formula necessary to determine your diet to reach the Zone is based on your individual protein needs and allocates a defined proportion of your daily food intake to carbohydrate and fat in proportion to your protein requirements, which are determined by a set of calculations involving your lean body mass (your weight and your percentage of body fat) and your activity level. All the calculations can be accomplished using the tools provided in his book, but they are complicated. This book is appropriate for anyone who is interested in athletics and enhancing physical performance.

Somers, Suzanne. *Eat Great, Lose Weight*. New York: Three Rivers Press, 1996.

Somers has developed an approach to weight loss and weight maintenance based on her own personal experience and food combining, the theory that different types of food need different environments to be properly digested. The proponents of this approach suggest that the stomach juices needed to digest meat are different from the stomach juices needed to digest carbohydrates. If we eat both types of food together, we do not properly digest either food and the result is indigestion, flatulence, and weight gain. Somers also suggests that there is too much natural sugar in fruits so they lose their nutritional value if eaten with anything else (the authors of *Fit for Life* have a slightly different theory). She maintains that if you want to eat fruit do so first thing in the morning then wait 30 to 90 minutes before eating anything else. If you have had a meal, you are advised to wait two to three hours before eating any fruit.

Somers's plan requires that you eliminate sugar, refined carbohydrates, caffeine, and alcohol in Level One. The rest of the allowable foods are divided into 1) Proteins and Fats, 2) Veggies, 3) Carbs, and 4) Fruits. Once you have sorted this out, there is a fairly detailed series of rules about eating and combining these food groups. For example, you may eat protein and fats with vegetables, or carbs with vegetables, but no fat. You must never combine proteins with carbs. In Level Two you are allowed to add small quantities of the foods eliminated in Level One. The basic rules of food combining remain unchanged. Although Somers provides recipes that include sugar (in reduced quantities) and flour, she readily admits that "In general, I find that the fewer carbs I eat, the more weight I lose" (p. 43). She does allow pasta, but never in combination with any protein or fats.

Somers's approach is not strictly low-carb or strict food combining, and while this combination has proved successful for her, we believe that it overcomplicates the issues. The book does provide a fascinating glimpse into the life of a famous personality, including family photos and personal vignettes. Anyone interested in her life, or in food combining principles, may want to read this book.

Willett, Walter C., MD. *Eat, Drink, and Be Healthy*. New York: Simon & Schuster, 2001.

In our opinion this is the best summary of the science available and is written in layperson's language, making it easy to understand. Dr. Willett is Chairman of the Harvard School of Public Health and a professor of medicine at Harvard Medical School. He is a world-renowned researcher, considered by many to be the preeminent nutritional epidemiologist in the world today. He sets the stage in the Introduction and then devotes a chapter to each major nutritional issue. He argues that the existing USDA Food Guide Pyramid is wrong. Instead of bread, cereal, rice, and pasta being the base of the pyramid with 6 to 11 servings per day, his Healthy Eating Pyramid puts these foods at the top of the pyramid, to be eaten sparingly. He also removes potatoes from the vegetable group.

Dr. Willett lists the seven healthiest changes you can make in your diet (pp. 22–24):

- Watch your weight.
- Eat fewer bad fats and more good fats.
- Eat fewer refined grain carbohydrates and more whole-grain carbohydrates.
- Choose healthier sources of proteins.
- Eat plenty of vegetables and fruits, but hold the potatoes.
- Use alcohol in moderation.
- Take a multivitamin for insurance.

Dr. Willett recommends physical activity, a diet that works for you, and becoming a defensive eater as the three most important factors in weight loss. Most of the suggestions offered by Dr. Willett are incorporated in our book, which is perhaps our highest compliment.

Articles from Scientific Literature

Bravata, Dena M., MD, MS, et al. "Efficacy and Safety of Low-Carbohydrate Diets: A Systematic Review." *Journal of the American Medical Association.* April 9, 2003, Vol. 2, No. 14, pages 1837–1850.

Bray, George A., MD., "Low-Carbohydrate Diets and Realities of Weight Loss." *Journal of the American Medical Association.* April 9, 2003, Vol. 2, No. 14, pages 1853–1855.

Curtis, Brian M., MD, and James H. O'Keefe, Jr., MD. "Understanding the Mediterranean Diet." *Postgraduate Medicine.* August 2002, Vol. 112, No. 2, pages 35–45.

Foster-Powell, Kaye, and Janette Brand Miller. "International Tables of Glycemic Index (GI)." *American Journal of Clinical Nutrition.* 1995, Vol. 62, No. 8, pages 71S–93S.

Hu, Frank B., MD, Ph.D. "The Mediterranean Diet and Mortality — Olive Oil and Beyond." *The New England Journal of Medicine.* June 26, 2003, Vol. 348, No. 26, pages 2595–2596.

Jenkins, David, et al. "Glycemic Index (GI) of Foods: A Physiological Basis for Carbohydrate Exchange." *The American Journal of Clinical Nutrition.* March 1981, Vol. 34, pages 362–66.

Mercola, Joseph, MD. "Managing Hypertriglyceridemia." *Canadian Medical Association Journal.* April 1, 2003, Vol. 168, No. 7, pages 831–32.

Michaud, D.S., et al. "Dietary Sugar, Glycemic Load (GL), and Pancreatic Cancer Risk." *Journal of the National Cancer Institute.* September 4, 2002, Vol. 94, No. 17, pages 1293–1300.

O'Keefe, James H. Jr., MD, and Loren Cordain, Ph.D. "How to Become a 21st Century Hunter-Gatherer — Cardiovascular Disease Resulting From a Diet and Lifestyle at Odds With Our Paleolithic Genome." *Mayo Clinic Proceedings.* 2004, Vol. 79, pages 101–108.

Sacks, Frank M., MD, and Matijn Katan, Ph.D. "Randomized Clinical Trials on the Effects of Dietary Fat and Carbohydrates on Plasma Lipoproteins and Cardiovascular Disease." *American Journal of Medicine.* December 30, 2002, Vol. 113, Supplement B.

Schwarz, J.M., P. Linfoot, D. Dare, and K. Aghajanian. "HighGrain Diet May Increase Risk of Cardiovascular Disease." *American Journal of Clinical Nutrition.* January 2003, Vol. 77, pages 43–50.

Trichopoulou, Antonia, et al. "Adherence to a Mediterranean Diet and Survival in a Greek Population." *The New England Journal of Medicine.* June 26, 2003, Vol. 348, No. 26, pages 2599–2608.

Westman, Eric, MD, et al. "Duke University Low-Carb Diet Research." *American Journal of Medicine.* July 2002, Vol. 113, No. 1, page 306.

Willett, Walter C., and Meir J. Stampfer. "Rebuilding the Food Pyramid." *Scientific American,* January 2003, pages 64–74.

Irene: Calgary, Alberta

It has been a great month. My husband and I were inspired by your radio broadcast and decided to try a low-carb approach again. We had tried the Atkins method two years ago, ignoring our food allergies completely. I actually lost little or no weight at all. Well, this time we are being true to our food allergies and have eliminated all wheat, dairy, and soy products. It is pretty challenging but the rewards are many. I also had been diagnosed as Type II Diabetes and am currently about 35 pounds overweight. I am able to control my sugar spikes with diet alone but am beginning to struggle more and more. I know that if the doctor were to test my A1C he would order me onto prescription drugs.

In our first month on low-carb I have lost 15 pounds and my sugar readings are consistently in the 5.0 to 7.0 range. I have so much energy I am able to finish everything I want to do each day. I no longer feel guilty. Before, by evening all of my energy was gone and I still had so much to do.

RECIPES

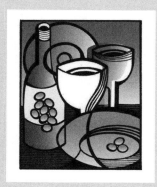

Contents

BREAKFAST FOODS

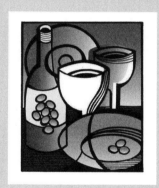

Baked Grapefruit

1 medium pink grapefruit
¼ teaspoon cinnamon
2 packets Splenda

- Preheat oven to 350°.
- Cut the grapefruit in half, and cut the sections with a grapefruit knife. Blend together the Splenda and cinnamon. Sprinkle the grapefruit halves with the spices.
- Place in a baking dish and bake for 20–25 minutes.
- Serve warm.

Makes 2 servings.

NOTE: This is a really exotic and delicious alternative to cold grapefruit. I always cut a small slice off each end to make a flat surface so that it sits better in the pan.

Nutrition Information Per Serving

Calories	45.71
Protein	0.82 g
Carbs	11.57 g
Fat	0.14 g
Fiber	1.56 g
Net carb	10.01 g

Breakfast Pie

1 teaspoon butter
¼ cup heavy cream
1 cup canned pumpkin (not the pie filling)
½ teaspoon Dijon mustard
¼ teaspoon paprika
½ teaspoon fresh ground pepper
6 eggs

• Preheat oven to 375°.
• Whisk eggs with cream and spices. Add Dijon mustard to pumpkin and blend into egg mixture with a fork.
• Bake in a buttered 9″ glass pie plate until browned, about 25–30 minutes.
Makes 6 servings.

NOTE: This is quite an unusual but tasty breakfast dish that can be reheated for lunch or dinner.

Nutrition Information Per Serving

Calories	134.02
Protein	7.91 g
Carbs	4.70 g
Fat	9.26 g
Fiber	0.02 g
Net carb	4.68 g

Easy Cheesy Quiche

6 eggs
½ cup light cream (half & half)
½ cup heavy cream
1 cup freshly shredded cheddar cheese
½ teaspoon fresh ground pepper
¼ teaspoon salt
½ tablespoon fresh chopped parsley

• Preheat oven to 375°.
• Whisk eggs, both creams, and salt & pepper,. Add the shredded cheese and blend gently with a fork.
• Pour into a buttered quiche dish or a 9″ pie plate.
• Bake for 25–30 minutes until lightly browned.
Makes 6 servings.

NOTE: This is also good reheated the following day for lunch or dinner.

Nutrition Information Per Serving

Calories	396.25
Protein	20.26 g
Carbs	4.27 g
Fat	32.95 g
Fiber	0.04 g
Net carb	4.23 g

Eggs Benedict

4 eggs
¼″ thick ham steak or small round ham
1 tablespoon olive oil
1 beefsteak tomato
½ cup Hollandaise Sauce (see recipe)
dash of paprika

- Heat olive oil in a frying pan over medium heat.
- Cut small ham into ¼″ slices, or cut ham steak into 3″ squares.
- Put ham in frying pan and brown on both sides. Remove from pan and place in a warm oven (approximately 250°).
- Cut tomato into ¼″ slices and cook in frying pan for just a minute or so on each side. Remove to warm oven.
- Poach 4 eggs for approximately 4 minutes. Eggs may be poached in the microwave, which will shorten cooking time, or in an electric poacher.
- To poach eggs in the frying pan, fill it with 1″ of water, crack the egg into a small dish or ramekin, and gently pour the egg into the boiling water to retain its shape. You may need to spoon the boiling water over the top of the yolk to ensure that it is properly cooked.
- To assemble the dish, place warm ham on the plate, then layer with cooked tomato and egg. Cover with warm Hollandaise Sauce. Sprinkle with paprika.

Makes 2 servings.

NOTE: This is a really delicious alternative to the other eggs Benedict. The most difficult part is the timing of the sauce and the eggs. An egg poacher goes a long way in simplifying the process.

Nutrition Information Per Serving

Calories	293.97
Protein	23.86 g
Carbs	4.99 g
Fat	19.10 g
Fiber	0.33 g
Net carb	4.66 g

Granola

....

1 cup All Bran Extra Fiber
1 cup rolled oats (not the instant variety)
½ cup soy nuts
½ cup slivered almonds
½ cup sunflower seeds
1 teaspoon cinnamon
¼ cup sugar-free syrup

- Preheat oven to 350°.
- Mix all ingredients together in a large bowl. Pour syrup over ingredients and stir to coat. Use just enough of any sugar-free syrup to allow mixture to bind. Place in a single layer on a cookie sheet covered with parchment paper.
- Bake for 25–30 minutes, stirring twice during the baking.
- Let cool completely and store in an airtight container.

Makes 4 cups of granola and 8 servings of ½cup each.

NOTE: This might seem like a lot of trouble, but it is a very tasty granola, and you can be sure of all the contents and the carb count. Make your own variety by adding a few raisins, some flax seed meal, or other nuts.

Nutrition Information Per Serving

Calories	174.39
Protein	11.35 g
Carbs	18.29 g
Fat	9.93 g
Fiber	10.22 g
Net carb	8.07 g

Hash Browns

2 tablespoons olive oil
2 cups cabbage, cut into 1″ pieces
¼ cup minced onion
1 cup pork rinds, roughly chopped
salt & ground pepper to taste

• Heat the olive oil over medium heat and add cabbage and onion. Sauté until tender, approximately 6–10 minutes.
• Add salt & pepper. Add the chopped pork rinds and continue to cook for 2 or 3 more minutes until everything is heated through and blended.
Makes 2 servings of approximately 1 cup each.

NOTE: This recipe calls for 1 cup of pork rinds before chopping or approximately 1/2 cup when chopped. The pork rinds add a really nice bacon flavor and some crispness to the dish. This is a great substitute for hash browns with breakfast.

Nutrition Information per Serving	
Calories	166.20
Protein	1.94 g
Carbs	9.73 g
Fat	14.70 g
Fiber	3.87 g
Net carb	5.86 g

Hollandaise Sauce

2 egg yolks
6 teaspoons butter
3 teaspoons lemon juice
⅛ teaspoon salt

- Place egg yolks and 2 teaspoons of butter in the top of a double boiler, over simmering water. Stir constantly with a whisk until butter melts.
- Add 2 teaspoons of butter and continue cooking. The sauce may start to thicken as you add the final 2 teaspoons of butter. Continue to cook and whisk until the butter is completely melted.
- Remove top of double boiler to a tea towel (to absorb any extra moisture) on nearby counter. Continue to whisk for 2 minutes. Add 3 teaspoons of lemon juice in 3 equal portions while whisking continuously.
- Add the salt and put back on top of double boiler for 2–3 minutes, until thickened, stirring constantly.
- If the sauce thickens too much, or starts to curdle, add 1–2 tablespoons of boiling water.

Makes approximately ½ cup of hollandaise sauce.

NOTE: This will make just enough for two servings of eggs Benedict that are not drowned in the sauce. The recipe may be doubled if you like lots of sauce.

Nutrition Information per Serving	
Calories	162.84
Protein	2.93 g
Carbs	0.80 g
Fat	16.66 g
Fiber	0.03 g
Net carb	0.77 g

Strawberry Smoothie

2 scoops (about 3 tablespoons) strawberry-flavored protein powder
½ cup frozen strawberries
¾ cup water

- Put all ingredients in a blender and process until smooth.

NOTE: If you want to cut your carb count, reduce the amount of frozen berries. Doing so will make the shake a little thinner in texture. You can also add just a tablespoon of heavy cream to add to the creamy texture of your shake.

Nutrition Information per Serving

Calories	86.08
Protein	10.32 g
Carbs	8.80 g
Fat	1.08 g
Fiber	2.56 g
Net carb	6.24 g

Sausage Pie

1 sausage (4–5 ounces)
6 large eggs
4 green onions, sliced
1 zucchini, quartered and cut into small pieces
½ red or green bell pepper, diced
½ cup light cream
1 cup shredded sharp cheddar cheese
1 teaspoon salt
½ teaspoon black pepper

• If the sausage has a casing, remove and discard it. Cut the sausage into bite-sized pieces. Cook the sausage in a large skillet until it crumbles
• Preheat oven to 325°.
• Add green onion, zucchini, and bell pepper and sauté until soft, about 5 minutes. Drain excess fat from dish.
• Whisk egg and light cream until blended. Add salt & pepper.
• In a lightly greased 9″ pie plate, place sausage and vegetable mixture, layer with cheese, and then pour egg mixture over all.
• At this point, you may cover and place the pie in the fridge overnight or for a few hours, or you may put the pie directly into the hot oven.
• Bake uncovered at 325° for 45–50 minutes if baking immediately, until edges are brown and egg is set. If taking out of the fridge, bake for 60 minutes.
Makes 6 servings.

NOTE: This is a great dish for breakfast, brunch, or lunch. Use any type of sausage, depending on your preferences.

Nutrition Information per Serving	
Calories	303.52
Protein	16.01 g
Carbs	5.47 g
Fat	23.83 g
Fiber	0.72 g
Net carb	4.75 g

Waffles

....

1 cup soy flour
1 tablespoon baking powder
3 packets Splenda
1 teaspoon salt
¼ cup heavy cream
¾ cup water
3 eggs
1 teaspoon vanilla

- Mix dry ingredients together in a bowl.
- Beat eggs until foamy in a separate bowl. Add remaining ingredients to eggs.
- Combine both wet and dry ingredients and mix well. This will make a very thick batter.
- Cook in a waffle iron, according to instructions.
- Serve with whipped cream, some jam (no sugar added), or fresh or frozen fruit.

Makes 6 waffles.

NOTE: The nutrition information was calculated for the waffles only. Be sure to calculate the additional carbs for whichever topping you choose.

TIP: If you do not have a waffle iron, you can make pancakes.

Thanks to Lynn Beach from Weyburn, Saskatchewan, for this recipe.

Nutrition Information per Serving	
Calories	154.56
Protein	9.70 g
Carbs	8.37 g
Fat	9.50 g
Fiber	2.67 g
Net carb	5.70 g

BREADS & MUFFINS

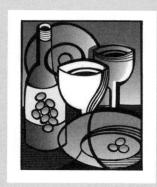

Basic Bread

1½ cups warm water
½ tablespoon active dry yeast
2 cups vital wheat gluten flour
1 egg
1 tablespoon olive oil
¼ teaspoon salt
1 tablespoon Splenda

- Add all ingredients in the order listed to your bread machine.
- Bake bread on the whole wheat setting on your machine. Set the crust setting to light if this option is available.

Makes approximately 10–12 slices.

NOTE: This bread can be made only with a bread machine because of the heavy elastic nature of the vital wheat gluten flour. This flour is high in protein and low in carbohydrates and can be found in the baking section of most grocery stores. Look for Bob's Red Mill brand, which is a popular variety of alternative flours and other baking ingredients. The recipe makes one decent-sized loaf.

Nutrition Information per Serving	
Calories	116.59
Protein	19.18 g
Carbs	5.13 g
Fat	17.31 g
Fiber	0.04 g
Net carb	5.09 g

NOTE: Nutrition information is based on a single slice, using 10 slices total for the loaf of bread.

Thanks to Joseph Gallacher of Victoria, British Columbia, for this tasty recipe, which inspired me to experiment with other varieties of low-carb breads.

Coconut Zucchini Muffins

½ cup ground almonds
¼ cup each ground sesame &
   sunflower seeds
½ cup flax seed meal
¼ cup soy flour
2 packets Splenda
½ teaspoon baking soda
½ teaspoon baking powder
½ teaspoon xanthan gum

¼ teaspoon salt
¼ cup sweetened coconut
1 egg, beaten
2 tablespoons olive oil
½ teaspoon coconut extract
¼ cup water
1 cup finely shredded zucchini
   (1 medium)

- Preheat oven to 375°.
- The nuts and seeds may be ground in a food processor.
- Mix all dry ingredients together. Mix wet ingredients in a separate bowl.
- Add wet ingredients to dry and stir to blend. Pour into muffin tins that have been lined with paper muffin cups.
- Bake for 25 minutes, until brown around the edges.

Makes 8 muffins.

VARIATION: You can substitute pumpkin seeds for the sesame seeds.

Many thanks to my sister Stephanie Tompkins for developing this recipe.

Nutrition Information per Serving

Calories	162.08
Protein	6.01 g
Carbs	5.43 g
Fat	13.85 g
Fiber	0.53 g
Net carb	4.90 g

Flax & Oat Bread

1¼ cups warm water
1 tablespoon olive oil
¼ teaspoon salt
1 egg
1 cup vital wheat gluten flour
½ cup flax seed meal
¼ cup oat flour
¼ cup soy flour
1 tablespoon Splenda
½ tablespoon active dry yeast

• Add all ingredients in the order listed to your bread machine.
• Bake bread on the whole wheat setting on your machine. Set the crust setting to light if this option is available.
Makes approximately 10–12 slices.

NOTE: This bread can only be made with a bread machine because of the heavy elastic nature of the vital wheat gluten flour. This flour is high in protein and low in carbohydrates and can be found in the baking section of most grocery stores. Look for Bob's Red Mill brand, which is a popular variety of alternative flours and other baking ingredients. The recipe makes one good-sized loaf.

Nutrition Information per Serving

Calories	74.80
Protein	9.50 g
Carbs	4.44 g
Fat	2.31 g
Fiber	0.69 g
Net carb	3.75 g

NOTE: Nutrition information is based on a single slice, using 10 slices total for the loaf of bread.

Flax & Oat Muffins

1 cup oat flour
½ cup soy flour
½ cup flax seed meal
½ teaspoon salt
2 teaspoons baking powder
⅔ cup light cream (half & half)
2 tablespoons olive oil
2 eggs

- Preheat oven to 425°.
- Mix all dry ingredients in a bowl.
- Whisk together eggs; then continue whisking as you add the other wet ingredients.
- Make a well in the dry ingredients, pour in the egg mixture, and mix thoroughly with a wooden spoon.
- Pour into a nonstick muffin pan.
- Bake for 15–18 minutes or until browned on top.

Makes 10 muffins.

VARIATION: These can be made into biscuits by dropping them on a nonstick cookie sheet and baking. For variety, try adding some bacon bits, chopped green onion, or dry herbs to the dough.

Nutrition Information per Serving

Calories	152.21
Protein	7.89 g
Carbs	11.60 g
Fat	8.90 g
Fiber	3.36 g
Net carb	8.24 g

Lemon Carrot Muffins

½ cup ground almonds
(or walnuts)
¼ cup each ground sesame and
sunflower seeds
½ cup flax seed meal
¼ cup soy flour
2 packets Splenda
½ teaspoon baking soda
½ teaspoon baking powder

½ teaspoon xanthan gum
¼ teaspoon salt
zest and juice of half a lemon
¼ cup raisins
1 egg, beaten
2 tablespoons olive oil
¼ cup plus 2 tablespoons water
1½ cups finely shredded carrot (2
medium)

• Preheat oven to 375°.
• The nuts and seeds may be ground in a food processor. The lemon zest needs to be very fine.
• Mix all dry ingredients together. Mix wet ingredients in a separate bowl.
• Add wet ingredients to dry and stir to blend. Pour into muffin tins that have been lined with paper muffin cups.
• Bake for 25 minutes, until brown around the edges.
Makes 8 muffins.

VARIATION: You may use orange juice and zest instead of lemon, but this will increase your carb count slightly. Substitute pumpkin seeds in place of sesame seeds.

Thanks again to my sister Stephanie Tompkins for developing this recipe.

Nutrition Information per Serving

Calories	169.77
Protein	6.12 g
Carbs	10.37 g
Fat	12.29 g
Fiber	1.40 g
Net carb	8.97 g

Magic Muffins

2 eggs, separated
5 tablespoons light olive oil
1 teaspoon vanilla
1 teaspoon baking powder
1 teaspoon cinnamon
¼ teaspoon nutmeg
2 packets Splenda
½ cup ground almonds
½ cup ground pecans
   (or walnuts)

1 cup flax seed meal
¼ cup whey (or soy) protein
   powder
1 cup finely shredded zucchini
1 cup finely shredded cabbage
½ cup finely shredded carrot
½ cup finely chopped
   cauliflower

• Preheat oven to 375°.
• Line a 12-medium-sized muffin tin with paper liners.
• Beat room temperature egg whites with a pinch of salt until stiff peaks form. Set aside.
• Finely shred and chop the vegetables, either by hand or in a food processor. Chop the nuts, or use a food processor on pulse for about 10 seconds. You do not want to pulverize the nuts, but they need to be very small. Combine the nuts and vegetables and blend well.
• Whisk together the egg yolks, olive oil, vanilla, cinnamon, nutmeg, Splenda, and baking powder until well mixed. Add the flax seed meal and the protein powder. This becomes a fairly dense mixture.
• Add the nuts and vegetables to the flax mixture and mix well. Fold in the egg white until blended.

continued

- Spoon the mixture into the lined muffin molds. Bake for 30–40 minutes, until nicely browned on top.

Makes 12 muffins.

VARIATION: You can vary the nuts to alter the flavor of these muffins. You may also substitute different vegetables, using yellow summer squash or broccoli, if desired. For the protein powder, you can use a vanilla or unflavored protein shake mix if you have one in your cupboard, or purchase one at the health food store. My friend Annette Wall suggested substituting savory seasonings for the cinnamon to make a savory muffin to have with soup.

Nutrition Information per Serving	
Calories	194.02
Protein	5.74 g
Carbs	7.60 g
Fat	16.75 g
Fiber	5.08 g
Net carb	2.52 g

Thanks to Valerie Caspersen of Victoria, British Columbia, who gave me the idea for these great muffins.

Oat Bran Bread

1 ¾ cups vital wheat gluten flour
2 tablespoons wheat bran
2 tablespoons oat bran
¼ cup flax seed meal
½ cup soy flour
1 tablespoon dry active yeast
1 tablespoon olive oil
½ cup water
2 eggs
½ teaspoon salt

- The water and eggs combined must equal 1 cup in total volume.
- Put all liquid ingredients in the bottom of a bread machine and add the salt.
- Mix all dry ingredients except the yeast in a large bowl and stir to blend. Put the dry ingredients into the bread maker. Make a well in the top and add the yeast.
- Set the bread maker to whole wheat setting, with a light crust if that is an option.
- This is a large and heavy loaf, and you will need a bread maker capable of a 2-pound loaf. It will give your machine a workout.
This loaf should provide 14 slices of bread.

NOTE: The nutrition information is calculated per slice.

Thanks to Bendt Caspersen of Victoria, British Columbia, for this recipe. Bendt notes that he does not have a bread maker but uses his Kitchen Aid mixer to mix the dough, lets the dough rise twice, and then bakes at 350° for an hour.

Nutrition Information per Serving	
Calories	108.00
Protein	15.66 g
Carbs	6.41 g
Fat	2.84 g
Fiber	1.13 g
Net carb	5.28 g

Oatmeal Flax Muffins

¾ cup vanilla whey protein
  powder
½ cup rolled oats
½ cup flax seed meal
2 tablespoons egg white powder
1 teaspoon baking powder
1 teaspoon cinnamon
½ teaspoon nutmeg
¼ teaspoon ground cloves
⅔ cup Splenda

⅛ teaspoon salt
½ cup canned pumpkin
1 tablespoon orange zest
¼ cup fresh orange juice
¼ cup water
¼ cup heavy cream
¼ cup chopped walnuts
3 large eggs
3 tablespoons olive oil

- Preheat oven to 350°.
- Spray a muffin pan with a nonstick agent and set aside.
- Mix all dry ingredients in a large bowl. The walnuts can be added after the other ingredients have been well blended.
- Whisk the eggs with the olive oil and then add the other wet ingredients, including the canned pumpkin, orange zest, and juice. It is easiest to add the pumpkin using a fork to blend.
- Make a well in the dry ingredients and pour the wet ingredients into the well. Blend well with a wooden spoon.
- Pour into the prepared muffin pan and bake for approximately 25–30 minutes, until edges are browned.

Makes 12 muffins.

VARIATION: You can substitute a 1/4 cup of raisins for the walnuts, although they will increase the carb content slightly.

Nutrition Information per Serving

Calories	139.71
Protein	5.80 g
Carbs	6.50 g
Fat	10.57 g
Fiber	2.34 g
Net carb	4.16 g

Oatmeal Pumpkin Muffins

1½ cups canned pumpkin, not the pie filling

1 teaspoon baking powder

1 teaspoon cinnamon

½ teaspoon nutmeg

¼ teaspoon ginger

¼ cup flax seed meal

½ cup vanilla whey protein

¼ cup oatmeal

9 packets Splenda

2 tablespoons egg white powder

¼ cup walnuts

¼ cup heavy cream

3 eggs

3 tablespoons olive oil

- Preheat oven to 375°.
- Spray muffin pan with a nonstick agent.
- Mix all dry ingredients in a bowl.
- In a separate bowl, whisk together eggs and oil. Add cream while continuing to whisk.
- Make a well in the dry ingredients. Add the wet ingredients and stir until well blended.
- Pour into prepared muffin pan and bake for 25–30 minutes, until brown at the edges.

Makes 12 muffins.

NOTE: Powdered egg white can be found in most health food stores.

Nutrition Information per Serving	
Calories	133.28
Protein	7.27 g
Carbs	5.86 g
Fat	9.69 g
Fiber	1.27 g
Net carb	4.59 g

Orange Cranberry Muffins

¾ cup vanilla whey protein
  powder
½ cup soy flour
½ cup flax seed meal
2 tablespoons egg white
  powder
1 teaspoon baking powder
¼ teaspoon ground ginger
½ teaspoon nutmeg
¼ teaspoon ground cloves

¼ cup Splenda
1 cup fresh cranberries,
  roughly chopped
zest & juice of a fresh
  orange
¼ cup water
¼ cup heavy cream
3 large eggs
3 tablespoons olive oil

- Preheat oven to 350°.
- Spray a muffin pan with a nonstick agent and set aside.
- Mix all dry ingredients in a large bowl.
- Whisk the eggs with the olive oil and then add the other wet ingredients, including the cranberries, orange zest, and juice.
- Make a well in the dry ingredients and pour the wet ingredients into the well. Blend well with a wooden spoon.
- Pour into the prepared muffin pan and bake for approximately 25–30 minutes, until edges are browned.

Makes 12 muffins.

VARIATION: You can substitute a 1/4 cup of dried cranberries for the fresh, although they will increase the carb content slightly. These muffins have a surprisingly pleasant tart note thanks to the cranberries. You will lose the tartness if you use the dried cranberries since they are much sweeter.

Nutrition Information per Serving	
Calories	151.72
Protein	10.94 g
Carbs	7.53 g
Fat	9.18 g
Fiber	2.61 g
Net carb	4.92 g

Raisin Flax Muffins

3 eggs

3 tablespoons butter

¼ cup water

3 tablespoons extra virgin olive oil

½ cup vanilla whey protein powder

2 tablespoons soy flour

2 teaspoons baking powder

3 tablespoons flax seed meal

6 packets Splenda

¼ cup raisins

• Preheat oven to 350°.
• Separate eggs and beat egg whites until they form stiff peaks.
• In a medium bowl, beat egg yolks with butter and olive oil and water.
• In a separate bowl, mix whey protein, soy flour, flax seed meal, raisins, Splenda, and baking powder.
• Beat dry mixture into egg yolk combination. Gently fold egg whites into batter and pour into a buttered nonstick muffin pan.
• Bake for 25–30 minutes, until inserted toothpick comes out clean.
Makes 8 muffins.

NOTE: If you want to reduce the carb content, reduce the amount of raisins.

Nutrition Information per Serving

Calories	178.68
Protein	7.40 g
Carbs	7.98 g
Fat	13.33 g
Fiber	1.85 g
Net carb	6.13 g

Walnut Flax Muffins

3 eggs, separated
3 tablespoons butter, melted
3 tablespoons light olive oil
½ cup vanilla whey protein powder
2 tablespoons soy flour
3 tablespoons flax seed meal
¼ cup walnuts, chopped
¼ cup water
½ teaspoon ground cinnamon
6 packets Splenda
2 teaspoons baking powder

- Separate eggs and beat egg whites until they form stiff peaks.
- In a medium bowl, whisk egg yolks with butter, olive oil, and water.
- In a separate bowl, sift whey protein, soy flour, cinnamon, Splenda, and baking powder. Add flax seed meal and walnuts and mix with a large wooden spoon.
- Blend dry mixture into egg yolk combination.
- Gently fold egg whites into batter and pour into a nonstick muffin pan that has been sprayed with a nonstick agent.
- Bake in a preheated oven at 350° for 25–30 minutes, until inserted toothpick comes out clean. The muffins will be golden brown on top with a slight sheen.
Makes 10 muffins.

Nutrition Information per Serving	
Calories	148.36
Protein	6.58 g
Carbs	3.78 g
Fat	12.37 g
Fiber	1.34 g
Net carb	2.44 g

Walnut Pumpkin Loaf

¾ cup vanilla whey protein powder

2 tablespoons egg white powder

1 tablespoon baking powder

1 teaspoon cinnamon

½ tablespoon ground cloves

½ teaspoon nutmeg

⅛ teaspoon mace

⅛ teaspoon ginger

⅔ cup Splenda

⅛ teaspoon salt

1½ cups canned pumpkin (not pie filling)

¼ cup heavy cream

¼ cup chopped walnuts

3 large eggs

3 tablespoons olive oil

2 tablespoons water

- Preheat oven to 375°.
- Spray a 9″ x 3″ x 5″ loaf pan with a nonstick agent and set aside.
- Mix all dry ingredients in a large bowl. The walnuts can be added after the other ingredients have been well blended.
- Whisk the eggs with the olive oil and then add the other wet ingredients, including the canned pumpkin. It is easiest to add the pumpkin using a fork to blend.
- Make a well in the dry ingredients and pour the wet ingredients into the well. Blend well with a wooden spoon.
- Pour into the prepared loaf pan and bake for approximately 1 hour and 10 minutes. Test with a toothpick.
- Let cool before cutting.

Makes approximately 12 slices.

NOTE: This is a wonderful midmorning or afternoon snack with a cup of tea.

My thanks to Louise Armstrong for inspiring this recipe.

Nutrition Information per Serving	
Calories	106.89
Protein	4.43 g
Carbs	4.53 g
Fat	8.28 g
Fiber	0.33 g
Net carb	4.20 g

Whole Wheat Flax Bread

1 cup and 2 tablespoons warm water
1 tablespoon olive oil
½ teaspoon salt
½ tablespoon dry active yeast
4 packets Splenda
1 cup vital wheat gluten flour
½ cup whole wheat flour
½ cup flax seed meal
½ cup wheat bran

• Place liquid ingredients in the bottom of a bread maker pan. Add the salt to the wet ingredients.
• Mix all dry ingredients, except the yeast, together in a bowl.
• Gently add the dry ingredients to the bread maker pan. Make a well in the top of the dry ingredients and add the yeast.
• Bake on the whole wheat setting, with a light crust if that is an option.
Makes a nice loaf with 12 slices of bread.

NOTE: This bread has a slightly higher carb count due to the whole wheat flour, but it is really delicious and worth the extra carbs once in a while. It is still well below any commercial breads in terms of carb content.

Nutrition Information per Serving

Calories	96.09
Protein	9.88 g
Carbs	9.15 g
Fat	3.87 g
Fiber	3.05 g
Net carb	6.10 g

APPETIZERS
& SNACKS

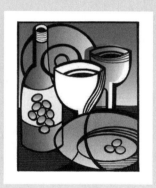

Cheese & Salmon Ball

6 ounces salmon, canned or
fresh cooked

8 ounces cream cheese

¼ cup red onion, minced

½ teaspoon chili powder

4 ounces cheddar cheese,
shredded

1 tablespoon sour cream

1 large egg, hard-boiled

¼ cup cashews

2 tablespoons chopped fresh
parsley

• Mix all ingredients except the nuts and parsley. It is easiest to do this with a
hand mixer, being careful not to purée the mixture.
• Divide the mixture into two equal parts. Place each batch into a small round
bowl, press down, and cover with plastic wrap. Place in the fridge for 2–3 hours.
• Invert the mixture onto the plastic wrap and use hands to even out any
irregularities in the ball. At this point, either one or both balls may be double-
wrapped and frozen. You may add the nuts before freezing, but leave the parsley
until just ready to serve as it does not freeze well.
• To finish, roughly chop nuts and parsley together. Place nut and parsley mixture on some wax paper and roll the cheese ball in the mixture, pressing lightly
to ensure that the nuts and parsley adhere.
Makes 2 balls of approximately 25–30 servings each.

NOTE: I serve these with fresh vegetables:
both carrot and celery sticks and cucumber
and zucchini rounds. Nutrition information
is calculated based on 50 servings of the
cheese & salmon ball only.

Thanks to Joseph Gallacher of Victoria,
British Columbia, for this delicious recipe.

**Nutrition Information
per Serving**

Calories	33.08
Protein	1.82 g
Carbs	0.53 g
Fat	2.67 g
Fiber	0.04 g
Net carb	0.49 g

Chocolate Nut Protein Bar

¼ cup soy protein powder

¼ cup unsalted peanuts

¼ cup pecans (or walnuts)

¼ cup almond slivers

¼ cup sunflower seeds

¼ cup pumpkin seeds

1 tablespoon oat flour

2 tablespoons unsweetened cocoa
   powder

6 packets Splenda

2 tablespoons whey protein powder

½ tablespoon xanthan gum

2–4 tablespoons water

1 teaspoon vanilla extract

2 tablespoons heavy cream

2 tablespoons olive oil

1 beaten egg

2 tablespoons peanut butter

2 tablespoons chocolate-flavored
   protein powder

- Preheat oven to 350°.
- Spray loaf pan with a nonstick agent.
- Put all dry ingredients in a food processor and blend well. (I leave a few pieces a bit bigger to provide texture and crunch.)
- Whisk egg and add olive oil, then water and cream. Finally, add peanut butter and vanilla to liquid and blend with whisk.
- Add dry ingredients to the wet and blend with a large spoon (use just enough water to allow you to blend the mixture). This will make a sticky and heavy batter.
- Place batter in loaf pan and spread evenly with the back of a spoon. Bake for 25 minutes, until golden brown at the edges.

Let cool.

Cut into 8 even bars.

NOTE: The flavor is somewhat dependent on the cocoa powder that you use. I use a rich dark cocoa powder. These freeze well.

Thanks to my sister Stephanie Tompkins, who did all the difficult preliminary work on these bars.

Nutrition Information per Serving	
Calories	222.91
Protein	9.56 g
Carbs	7.32 g
Fat	18.26 g
Fiber	0.89 g
Net carb	6.43 g

Citrus Protein Bar

¼ cup soy protein powder

1 teaspoon cinnamon

1 teaspoon nutmeg

¼ cup pecans (or walnuts)

¼ cup almond slivers

¼ cup sunflower seeds

¼ cup pumpkin seeds

¼ cup unsweetened coconut

4 packets Splenda

3 tablespoons whey protein powder

1 tablespoon xanthan gum

¼ cup water

zest of 1 lemon

2 tablespoons light cream

2 tablespoons olive oil

1 beaten egg

2 tablespoons no-sugar-added apricot jam

• Preheat oven to 350°.
• Spray loaf pan with a nonstick agent.
• Put all dry ingredients in a food processor and blend well. (I leave a few pieces a bit bigger to provide texture and crunch.)
• Whisk egg and add olive oil, then water and light cream. Finally, add jam and fine lemon zest to liquid and blend with whisk.
• Add dry ingredients to the wet and blend with a large spoon. This will make a sticky and heavy batter.
• Place batter in loaf pan and spread evenly with the back of a spoon. Bake for 25 minutes, until golden brown at the edges.

Let cool.

Cut into 8 even bars.

VARIATION: Change the flavor with different jams. E.D. Smith makes a strawberry and a blackberry no-sugar-added jam that would be nice in these bars.

Thanks to my sister Stephanie Tompkins, who did all the difficult preliminary work on these bars.

Nutrition Information per Serving	
Calories	177.47
Protein	7.21 g
Carbs	5.44 g
Fat	14.94 g
Fiber	0.96 g
Net carb	4.48 g

Crab Dip

1 package (250 grams) Philadelphia Cream Cheese

1 can (120 grams) crab meat

1 cup mayonnaise

1 tablespoon Sambal Oelek (hot chili sauce)

½ cup finely shredded cheddar cheese

- Preheat oven to 350°.
- Cut Philadelphia cheese into chunks and place in an oven-proof dish (either 1.5- or 2-quart dish). Place a cover on the dish and heat the cheese in the oven for approximately 15 minutes.
- While the cheese is in the oven, mix the crab meat with the mayonnaise and the hot chili sauce until well blended.
- Remove the cheese from the oven and add the crab mixture. Mix well and scrape down the sides of the dish with a spatula.
- Replace the dish, still covered, in the oven for 20 minutes. Then remove from the oven and sprinkle the grated cheddar cheese on top and put back in the oven, uncovered, for 5–10 minutes, until the cheese is melted and the crab mixture is brown at the edges.
- Serve warm or cold with fresh veggies for dipping.

Makes approximately 48 servings of 2 teaspoons each.

VARIATION: Use shredded Swiss cheese. This will be a slightly more subtle taste addition, and the color will blend well with the crab. Another variation might be to add a little more of the hot chili sauce, depending on your taste buds. As it appears here, it has a nice little afterbite!

NOTE: You will probably find the Sambal Oelek, a hot chili sauce, in the Chinese-cooking section of your grocery store.

Nutrition Information per Serving	
Calories	50.33
Protein	1.29 g
Carbs	0.39 g
Fat	4.89 g
Fiber	0.00 g
Net carb	0.39 g

Thanks to Joanne Francis of Delta, British Columbia, for this delicious recipe.

Glazed Walnuts

3 cups walnuts
4 packets Splenda
1 teaspoon paprika
½ teaspoon cayenne
½ teaspoon nutmeg
¼ cup soy sauce
1 tablespoon butter

- Preheat oven to 250°.
- Melt butter and mix with soy sauce, Splenda, and spices. Place nuts in a large bowl and pour butter and spice mixture over nuts. Stir to coat.
- Line a cookie sheet with parchment paper. Arrange nuts in a single layer on cookie sheet. Use a rubber spatula to scrape bowl and pour any leftover sauce on the walnuts.
- Bake for approximately 30–35 minutes or until brown. Stir a couple of times while baking. Immediately loosen the nuts with a spatula before allowing them to cool. Place in an airtight container.

Makes 24 servings of 2 tablespoons each.

NOTE: These are great as snacks or sprinkled over some ice cream.

Nutrition Information per Serving

Calories	89.03
Protein	2.10 g
Carbs	2.15 g
Fat	8.67 g
Fiber	0.88 g
Net carb	1.27 g

Party Nuts

2 egg whites
1 cup unsalted almonds
1 cup unsalted walnuts
1 cup unsalted pecans
1 cup unsalted peanuts
8 packets Splenda
1 teaspoon cinnamon
1 teaspoon cayenne pepper
½ teaspoon salt
¼ teaspoon nutmeg

- Preheat oven to 325°.
- Whisk the egg whites with the salt until foamy.
- Put the Splenda and the spices in a small bowl and blend together.
- Put the nuts in a large bowl, pour the foamy egg whites over them, and stir to coat. Sprinkle the spices over the nuts and stir well.
- Spray a cookie sheet with a nonstick agent. Spread the nuts evenly on the cookie sheet and place in the oven for approximately 15–20 minutes, until browned. The nuts need to be stirred frequently to keep from burning.
- Cool and store in an airtight container.

Makes 4 cups.

NOTE: Nutrition information is calculated on a serving size of 1/5 cup.

Nutrition Information per Serving

Calories	159.38
Protein	4.33 g
Carbs	5.67 g
Fat	14.41 g
Fiber	1.90 g
Net carb	3.77 g

Salmon Ball

1 can (7.5 ounces) salmon
1 package (250 grams) cream cheese
1 tablespoon fresh lemon juice
1 green onion, finely chopped
1½ tablespoons horseradish
¼ teaspoon paprika

Topping
⅔ cup chopped walnuts
¼ cup chopped fresh parsley
2 tablespoons chopped fresh dill

- Cream together first six ingredients with a whisk, until smooth.
- Place the salmon mixture in a small cereal bowl. Cover with plastic wrap and press the wrap down to the surface of the salmon. Make a tight package. Place in the fridge overnight or for at least 2–3 hours.
- Mix together the ingredients for the topping in a large bowl.
- Remove the salmon ball from the bowl and roll it in the topping, pressing firmly.
- Place the ball on a serving plate and garnish with fresh dill stems. Serve with sliced cucumber or small low-carb crackers.

Makes approximately 2 cups.

NOTE: Nutrition information is based on 100 servings of approximately 1 teaspoon each and does not include the crackers or cucumber slices.

Thanks to my sisters, Stephanie Tompkins and Kathy Spampinato, each of whom provided ideas for this recipe.

Nutrition Information per Serving

Calories	15.96
Protein	1.14 g
Carbs	0.18 g
Fat	1.22 g
Fiber	0.03 g
Net carb	0.15 g

Spicy Southern Pecans

3 cups raw pecan halves
1 large egg white
½ cup Splenda
1 tablespoon paprika
1 teaspoon cayenne pepper
½ teaspoon cinnamon
½ teaspoon nutmeg
2 teaspoons Worcestershire Sauce

- Preheat oven to 250°.
- Whisk the egg white until frothy.
- Mix the spices with the Splenda in a small bowl and blend well.
- Add the Worcestershire Sauce to the egg white and then the spices, mixing until well blended.
- Add the nuts to the egg white mixture and mix well to coat.
- Spread nuts in a single layer on a baking sheet lined with parchment paper. Pour any remaining egg mixture over nuts.
- Bake for 1–11/4 hours, until the nuts are completely dry. Stir the nuts every 20 minutes to bake evenly.

Makes 24 servings of 2 tablespoons each.

NOTE: We love these nuts, but save them for Christmas and other special occasions because it is hard not to eat them all at once.

Nutrition Information per Serving	
Calories	97.97
Protein	1.53 g
Carbs	2.74 g
Fat	9.87 g
Fiber	1.41 g
Net carb	1.33 g

Tuna Cheese Dip

8 ounces cream cheese, softened
6-ounce can of white tuna
2 tablespoons Sambal Oelek (chili sauce)
2 tablespoons dried parsley
2 tablespoons finely minced onion
salt & white pepper, to taste
¼ cup chopped walnuts to garnish

• Mix all ingredients (except the walnuts) with a fork until well blended. Mold into a ball in the bottom of a bowl, cover with plastic wrap, and chill in the fridge for at least 2 hours.
• Remove from bowl and roll the ball in the chopped nuts.
• Serve with fresh vegetables such as sliced zucchini and cucumber or celery and carrot sticks.

Makes 48 servings of approximately 1 teaspoon each.

NOTE: This delicious dip may also be made with shrimp or crab meat. Sambal Oelek is a ground red chili paste that you can find in the Chinese-cooking section of a grocery store.

Thanks to Nancy Cieminski of Winona, Minnesota, for this great recipe.

Nutrition Information per Serving	
Calories	20.70
Protein	1.21 g
Carbs	0.16 g
Fat	1.73 g
Fiber	0.01 g
Net carb	0.15 g

SOUPS & SALADS

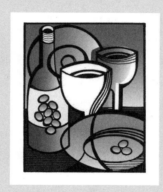

Cauliflower & Cheddar Soup

1 medium cauliflower (about 1½ pounds)
1 garlic clove, minced
1 tablespoon chopped fresh thyme
4 cups chicken broth
1 cup light cream (half & half)
1 teaspoon cornstarch
1½ cups grated sharp white cheddar cheese
½ cup finely chopped green onion
¼ teaspoon salt
freshly ground pepper, to taste

• Cut the cauliflower into small florets. Place them in a soup pot with the garlic, thyme, and chicken broth. Bring to a boil and reduce the heat to simmer and cook until the cauliflower is soft, about 10 minutes.
• Whisk the cornstarch into the light cream until dissolved. Slowly pour into the pot, stirring constantly.
• Remove the pot from the heat and remove ¾ of the soup and blend in a food processor or blender. Return the puréed soup to the soup pot with the reserved florets. Simmer, stirring occasionally, for 5–10 minutes, until the soup is slightly thickened.
• Gradually add the grated cheese, stirring constantly, until it is melted. Add the salt, pepper to taste, and green onion, reserving a few slices for garnish.
Makes 6 servings.

Nutrition Information per Serving	
Calories	226.36
Protein	12.40 g
Carbs	7.15 g
Fat	17.08 g
Fiber	1.81 g
Net carb	5.34 g

Cheesy Cabbage Soup

1 small onion, minced
1 tablespoon olive oil
1 garlic clove, minced
5 cups chicken broth
2½ cups coarsely chopped cabbage
½ cup shredded Swiss cheese
½ cup shredded white cheddar cheese
1 cup cooked ham, cubed
1 teaspoon cornstarch
1 cup heavy cream
1 cup grated carrot
1 tablespoon chopped fresh parsley
¼ teaspoon salt
freshly ground pepper, to taste

• In a large saucepan or soup pot, sauté the onion and garlic in the olive oil until just soft. Do not brown. Pour in the chicken broth, add the cabbage, parsley, and carrot, and bring to a boil. Reduce heat and simmer for 10 minutes.
• Dissolve the cornstarch in the heavy cream and add to the soup pot, stirring constantly. Gradually stir in the cheese until melted. Add the cubed ham and salt & pepper, to taste. Simmer for an additional 5 minutes, stirring occasionally.
Makes 6 servings.

Nutrition Information per Serving	
Calories	318.24
Protein	13.64 g
Carbs	7.39 g
Fat	26.54 g
Fiber	1.46 g
Net carb	5.93 g

Chunky Ham Soup

1 cup diced cooked ham
2 tablespoons light olive oil
2 garlic cloves, minced
1½ tablespoons chopped fresh parsley
1 medium sweet onion, minced
8 cups chicken or beef stock
4 large celery sticks, cut into ½" pieces
1 cup sliced mushrooms
2 cups sliced cabbage
1 cup trimmed green beans
1 cup asparagus spears, cut into 1" pieces
1 medium carrot, thinly sliced

• Heat olive oil over medium heat in a large soup pot. Add the onion and garlic and sauté for about 3–4 minutes. Add the mushrooms and parsley and continue cooking for 3 or 4 more minutes, until the mushrooms are soft.
• Add the chicken (or beef) stock and the cabbage, beans, carrots, and cauliflower. Simmer for approximately 1 hour.
• Add the diced ham, asparagus, and celery and continue to simmer for 15 minutes.
Makes 4 servings.

TIP: This soup may be refrigerated and reheated before serving.

Nutrition Information per Serving	
Calories	202.90
Protein	12.13 g
Carbs	10.99 g
Fat	13.34 g
Fiber	4.02 g
Net carb	6.97 g

French Onion Soup

1 pound onions (4 cups sliced)
¼ cup butter
3 cloves garlic, minced
6 cups beef bouillon
½ teaspoon salt
freshly ground pepper, to taste
1½ cups shredded mozzarella

- Mince the garlic and cut whole, peeled onions into thin rounds.
- Melt butter in a large soup pot and add the onion and garlic. Caramelize the onion by cooking it over medium heat until the natural sugar is released and the onion turns brown and is reduced in volume. This will take about 25–30 minutes, during which time the mixture should be stirred frequently.
- Add the beef bouillon and salt & freshly ground black pepper; then reduce heat and simmer for 35 minutes.
- To serve, pour the soup into 4 oven-proof soup bowls. Sprinkle each bowl with shredded cheese, and place all 4 bowls on a cookie sheet.
- Place the cookie sheet under a hot broiler for 2–3 minutes, until the cheese is melted and has browned.

Makes 4 servings.

NOTE: If you are worried about the fat content of this soup, reduce the amount of shredded cheese that you use for finishing the soup.

Thanks to my sister Kathy Spampinato, who provided the basic recipe for this soup.

Nutrition Information Per Serving	
Calories	359.76
Protein	20.58 g
Carbs	10.58 g
Fat	26.66 g
Fiber	1.41 g
Net carb	9.17 g

Hearty Vegetable Soup

2 tablespoons light olive oil
2 cloves garlic, minced
1½ tablespoons chopped fresh parsley
1 medium sweet onion, minced
8 cups chicken or beef stock
4 large celery sticks, cut into ½" pieces
1 cup sliced mushrooms
2 cups sliced cabbage
1 cup trimmed green beans
1 cup asparagus spears, cut into 1" pieces
1 cup cauliflower florets
1 medium zucchini, cut into ½" pieces
1 medium carrot, thinly sliced

• Heat olive oil over medium heat in a large soup pot. Add the onion and garlic and sauté for about 3–4 minutes. Add the mushrooms and parsley and continue cooking for 3 or 4 more minutes, until the mushrooms are soft.
• Add the chicken (or beef) stock and the cabbage, beans, carrots, and cauliflower. Simmer for approximately 1 hour.
• Add the asparagus, celery, and zucchini and continue to simmer for 15 minutes.
Makes 4 servings.

TIP: This soup may be refrigerated and reheated before serving.

Nutrition Information per Serving	
Calories	117.89
Protein	3.78 g
Carbs	12.16 g
Fat	7.52 g
Fiber	4.85 g
Net carb	7.31 g

Meatball Soup

1–1½ pounds extra lean ground
   beef
1 egg
2 tablespoons bread crumbs
½ teaspoon ground black
   pepper
¼ teaspoon salt

2 tablespoons olive oil
½ cup diced onion
1 cup sliced mushrooms
4 cups chopped cabbage
2 cloves garlic, minced
3 medium carrots, chopped
6 cups beef broth

• Combine the ground beef with beaten egg, bread crumbs, and salt & pepper.
• Heat olive oil over medium heat in a large soup pot. Form beef mixture into ½″ balls and brown on all sides. You may have to do this in lots, depending on the size of your pot. Remove meatballs and set aside.
• Add onion and mushrooms and sauté for 5 minutes or until soft. Be sure to scrape the bottom of the pan to loosen any brown bits since they add to the flavor. Add ½ cup of the beef broth and continue to work away at the brown bits on the bottom.
• Add the remaining 5½ cups of beef broth into the pot. Carefully add the meatballs back into the pot. Stir in the chopped carrots and cabbage. You may want to add a little extra freshly ground pepper & salt at this point. Reduce heat and simmer, covered, for 1 or 2 hours.
Makes 6–8 servings.

NOTE: Nutrition information is calculated based on 1 1/2 pounds of ground beef and 6 servings of soup.

Thanks to Mary Sinclair of Thunder Bay, Ontario, who provided the inspiration for this soup.

Nutrition Information per Serving	
Calories	329.21
Protein	26.18 g
Carbs	9.69 g
Fat	20.77 g
Fiber	2.67 g
Net carb	7.02 g

Tomato, Herb, & Curried Chicken Soup

2 boneless, skinless chicken breasts

3 tablespoons extra virgin olive oil

¼ teaspoon mustard seeds

¼ teaspoon ground cumin

2 teaspoons curry powder

¼ cup heavy cream

4 cloves garlic, minced

½ sweet onion, minced

1 cup chicken bouillon

4 large, ripe tomatoes, roughly chopped

4 packets Splenda

2 tablespoons chopped fresh flat leaf parsley

2 tablespoons chopped fresh rosemary

1 tablespoon chopped fresh chives

fresh chives for garnish

freshly ground pepper

• Heat 2 tablespoons of olive oil in a soup pot or large stew pot. Add the minced onion and garlic and sauté for 2–3 minutes. Add the fresh herbs and continue cooking for 1 minute.

• Add the tomatoes (these should be roughly chopped into 1″ pieces) and Splenda and simmer, stirring frequently, for approximately 15–20 minutes, until cooked through and soft.

• Prepare the chicken while the tomatoes are simmering. Cut the chicken into ½″ pieces.

continued

- Heat 1 tablespoon of the olive oil in a nonstick frying pan. Add the chicken and sauté over medium heat until browned on all sides. Remove chicken from the pan and set aside.
- Add the mustard seed, cumin, and curry to the pan. Add the heavy cream and stir to blend. Add back the chicken with any juices and stir for a minute to coat. Turn off heat and set aside.
- Take approximately ¾ of the tomato mixture, put it into a food processor, and blend until smooth.
- Return the tomato mixture to the soup pot and add the chicken bouillon, stirring to blend. You now have a mostly creamy tomato base, with a few chunky pieces to add texture.
- Add the chicken with the curry sauce to the soup, stirring to blend the sauce with the soup. Season with freshly ground pepper and simmer for 15 minutes to allow the flavors to blend.
- Serve with a couple of fresh chives floating on the soup and a sprinkle of freshly ground pepper.

Makes 4 servings.

NOTE: The inspiration for this really delicious soup came from a lovely country inn just outside Queenstown, New Zealand. I thought about this soup for months, making constant notes, before trying to put it together. It took more than a couple of trials, but the result is well worth it, I think.

Nutrition Information per Serving	
Calories	163.75
Protein	13.82 g
Carbs	5.42 g
Fat	8.97 g
Fiber	1.44 g
Net carb	3.98 g

Turkey Broth

1 turkey carcass
4–5 quarts water
1 onion, quartered
1 carrot, cut up
6 celery tops with leaves
salt & pepper, to taste

- Place the carcass in a large soup or stew pot with sufficient water to cover the carcass.
- Add the carrot, onion, and celery tops. Cover pot and simmer for 2–3 hours.
- Strain the broth 2 or 3 times to eliminate the bones, vegetables, and other bits.
- Cool in the fridge overnight. Remove from fridge and skim off any fat that may have solidified on top.

Makes 4–5 quarts of turkey broth, depending on size of carcass and amount of water used.

NOTE: Nutrition calculation is for the entire batch of broth. Make your own chicken broth using essentially the same recipe and substituting one or more chicken carcasses.

Nutrition Information per Serving	
Calories	117.77
Protein	14.34 g
Carbs	2.39 g
Fat	5.33 g
Fiber	0.57 g
Net carb	1.82 g

Turkey Soup

3–4 quarts turkey broth (see previous page)
1 medium sweet onion, minced
6–8 medium carrots, thinly sliced
2 cups cauliflower florets
2 cups green beans, cut into ½" pieces
4 cups green cabbage, cut into 1" pieces
2 cups chopped celery
4 cups bite-sized cooked turkey meat
salt & freshly ground pepper, to taste

• Pour turkey broth into a large soup pot with a lid. Add prepared vegetables and salt & pepper.
• Simmer, covered, for at least 2 hours. The cauliflower will break up and become almost like barley. The cabbage replaces rice and provides extra bulk and flavor.
• One hour before serving, add the turkey meat, cover, and continue to simmer. Taste for seasoning at this point and add more salt & pepper if needed.
Makes 8–10 servings.

NOTE: This is a delicious, filling soup. It is a meal on its own. The soup freezes well or will stay fresh in the fridge for a couple of days.

Nutrition Information per Serving	
Calories	200.69
Protein	19.90 g
Carbs	12.96 g
Fat	7.77 g
Fiber	4.03 g
Net carb	8.93 g

Curried Mango Salad

6 cups mixed greens
1 ripe mango, diced
½ cup whole roasted cashews
2 chopped green onions
Curried Red Wine Dressing (see recipe)

• Wash and wipe dry all greens. Add mango and onion to the greens. Keep cashews in a separate small dish until ready to dress.

• Dress the salad with the Curried Red Wine Dressing just before serving.
Makes 6 servings if used as an appetizer or 4 lunch-sized servings.

NOTE: Nutrition information is calculated based on 6 servings.

TIP: To reduce the grams of carbohydrates, use just half a mango. This fruit is delicious but high in carbs. You can also substitute papaya for the mango to reduce the carb content. I always use fresh baby spinach as part of my greens to increase the fiber in the salad.

Nutrition Information per Serving	
Calories	270.40
Protein	4.98 g
Carbs	13.74 g
Fat	23.28 g
Fiber	3.90 g
Net carb	9.84 g

Thanks to my good friend Jacqueline McDonald of Toronto, Ontario, for this recipe, which I adapted slightly.

Egg Salad

4 hard-boiled eggs
1 celery stick, finely minced
1 green onion, finely chopped
¼ cup red or green pepper, finely minced
⅔ cup mayonnaise
1½ teaspoons Dijon mustard
½ teaspoon salt
freshly ground pepper, to taste
6–8 red lettuce leaves

• Place 4 eggs in a pot and cover with water. Bring to a boil, reduce heat, and boil for 10 minutes. Rinse the eggs in cold water to cool them and place them in the fridge for at least an hour.
• Crack the eggshells and peel off. Roughly chop the eggs. Add the celery, onion, and red or green pepper.
• Mix the mayonnaise, mustard, and salt & pepper. Add the dressing to the egg mixture and mix gently until just blended.
• Serve on a bed of red lettuce.
Makes 2–3 servings.

Nutrition Information Per Serving	
Calories	293.68
Protein	9.61 g
Carbs	2.79 g
Fat	28.04 g
Fiber	0.46 g
Net carb	2.33 g

Grapefruit & Spinach Salad

1 pound fresh baby spinach (about 8 cups)
2 fresh pink grapefruits
½ cup toasted almond slivers
Creamy White Wine Vinaigrette (see recipe)

• Wash the spinach and remove stems. Place on paper towels to dry. Tear into bite-sized pieces and place in a large bowl.
• Peel the grapefruit and separate into natural sections. Peel the sections and cut into ½" pieces.
• Add the grapefruit to the spinach and toss. Add the almonds and dressing just before serving.
Makes 4 lunch-sized servings or 6 appetizer salads.

NOTE: Nutrition calculation is based on 6 servings. This is a delicious new twist on a spinach salad. It is great as an appetizer at dinner or as a lunch salad.

Nutrition Information per Serving	
Calories	103.60
Protein	4.25 g
Carbs	9.96 g
Fat	6.34 g
Fiber	3.24 g
Net carb	6.72 g

Marinated Veggies

2 cups broccoli florets
2 cups cauliflower florets
1 English cucumber with peel, quartered and sliced
2 cups celery, diced
1 medium sweet red pepper, chopped
1 medium sweet yellow pepper, chopped
1 cup carrot, sliced or julienned
Creamy Vegetable Marinade (see recipe)

- Wash, pat dry, and cut all vegetables.
- Put vegetables in a large bowl and pour marinade over them. Stir well to coat. Place in fridge for at least a couple of hours before serving.
Makes 8 servings.

VARIATION: This is a great salad that can have many variations by adding any vegetable you like. Keep in mind that some veggies have more carbs than others. To keep your carb content down, add asparagus, green onions, mushrooms, or green beans.

NOTE: This salad will keep for 2–3 days in an airtight container in the fridge.

Nutrition Information per Serving

Calories	167.26
Protein	2.19 g
Carbs	9.15 g
Fat	14.44 g
Fiber	2.34 g
Net carb	6.81 g

Oriental Chicken Salad

2 cooked boneless chicken breasts (use Orange Chicken)
4 cups shredded iceberg lettuce
4 cups chopped or shredded green cabbage
4 small green onions, chopped
1 cup chopped or shredded bok choy
½ small sweet red pepper, thinly sliced
1 cup bean sprouts
½ cup mandarin orange pieces
½ cup toasted almond slivers
1 teaspoon sesame seeds, to garnish
Soy Ginger Dressing (see recipe)

• Roughly chop lettuce, cabbage, and bok choy and place in a large bowl. Slice green onion and red pepper and add to bowl.
• Cut cooked chicken into bite-sized pieces and set aside.
• Add mandarin orange sections to bowl, along with roasted almond slivers and bean sprouts. Mix all ingredients.
• Toss the salad with Soy Ginger Dressing.
• Divide the salad evenly among 4 plates. Place chicken pieces on top and sprinkle with sesame seeds.
Makes 4 servings.

Nutrition Information per Serving	
Calories	333.60
Protein	37.84 g
Carbs	17.19 g
Fat	10.94 g
Fiber	5.61 g
Net carb	11.58 g

Oriental Coleslaw

1 cup green cabbage, chopped
3 cups napa cabbage, chopped
2 cups red cabbage, chopped
1 carrot, grated
½ cup thinly sliced red onion
Oriental Dressing (see recipe)

- Wash and cut all vegetables and combine in a large bowl.
- Toss the slaw with the dressing, cover, and chill in the fridge for an hour to allow the flavors to blend.

Makes 6–8 servings.

NOTE: Nutrition information is calculated based on 8 servings. This is a really fun and tasty variation on coleslaw. The hot note in the dressing is a surprise. As with the other varieties, it will keep well in the fridge for 2–3 days.

TIP: To prevent the red color from running, rinse the sliced red cabbage under cold water in a colander, until the water runs clear.

Nutrition Information per Serving	
Calories	99.51
Protein	1.40 g
Carbs	6.69 g
Fat	8.21 g
Fiber	1.89 g
Net Fiber	4.80 g

Salmon & Avocado Salad

juice of half a lemon
2 ripe avocados
2 chopped green onions
½ cup diced celery
½ cup diced red pepper
1 can (7.5 ounces) of salmon (or cooked fresh salmon if available)
2 tablespoons mayonnaise
¼ teaspoon salt
chopped fresh dill

- Squeeze half a lemon and put juice in a bowl.
- Cut avocados in half lengthwise and dispose of pits. Scoop avocado out of the shells and set shells aside. Dice the avocado into very small pieces and place pieces in lemon juice. Stir well to coat to prevent browning.
- Add the green onion, celery, and red pepper.
- Mash the salmon well (including bones, if you like) and add to the avocado mixture. Add salt and chopped fresh dill, to taste.
- Add the mayonnaise and stir well.
- Fill the avocado half shells and sprinkle on some chopped dill to garnish.

Makes 4 appetizer servings or 2 lunch servings.

VARIATION: This salad may also be made with crab meat.

NOTE: Nutrition information is calculated based on 4 servings.

Thanks to our good friend Donna Jones from Nova Scotia for this great recipe.

Nutrition Information per Serving	
Calories	284.01
Protein	12.32 g
Carbs	8.86 g
Fat	24.16 g
Fiber	4.90 g
Net carb	3.96 g

Spinach & Strawberry Salad

6 cups spinach, raw
1 cup sliced strawberries
½ cup toasted almond slivers
¼ cup thinly sliced red onion
Red Wine Vinaigrette (see recipe)

- Toast the almond slivers until lightly browned.
- Wash and pat dry the spinach. Tear off stems and tear leaves into bite-sized pieces.
- Wash and pat dry the strawberries. Slice into thin pieces down the sides to show the shape of the berries.
- Combine all ingredients in a large bowl and toss with Red Wine Vinaigrette. *Makes 4 servings.*

Nutrition Information per Serving

Calories	130.39
Protein	5.60 g
Carbs	8.72 g
Fat	9.50 g
Fiber	4.18 g
Net carb	4.54 g

SALAD DRESSINGS

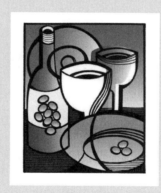

Balsamic Vinaigrette

¼ cup olive oil
⅔ cup balsamic vinegar
1 teaspoon dry mustard
1 teaspoon chopped fresh parsley
1 packet Splenda
½ teaspoon freshly ground pepper

• Whisk together the vinaigrette ingredients.
Makes enough dressing for 4 servings.

Nutrition Information per Serving	
Calories	135.57
Protein	0.03 g
Carbs	3.37 g
Fat	14.03 g
Fiber	0.04 g
Net carb	3.33 g

Creamy Dijon Vinaigrette

¾ cup extra virgin olive oil

⅓ cup red wine vinegar

1 tablespoon Dijon mustard

1 clove garlic, minced

2 teaspoons Worcestershire Sauce

2 packets Splenda

¼ teaspoon ground black pepper

⅛ teaspoon salt

• Put all ingredients in a blender and blend until well combined.
Makes 8 servings of 2 tablespoons each.

Nutrition Information per Serving

Calories	188.54
Protein	0.40 g
Carbs	1.29 g
Fat	21.40 g
Fiber	0.05 g
Net carb	1.24 g

Creaky Raspberry Vinaigrette

½ cup extra virgin olive oil

⅔ cup raspberry vinegar

1 teaspoon Dijon mustard

1 packet Splenda

⅛ teaspoon salt

2 teaspoons chopped fresh parsley

• Put all ingredients in a blender and blend until well combined.
Makes 6 servings of 2 tablespoons each.

Nutrition Information per Serving	
Calories	169.17
Protein	0.40 g
Carbs	1.53 g
Fat	19.07 g
Fiber	0.03 g
Net carb	1.50 g

Creamy White Wine Vinaigrette

⅔ cup extra virgin olive oil

3 tablespoons white wine vinegar

1 teaspoon Dijon mustard

1 clove garlic, minced

1 teaspoon dried parsley

1 packet Splenda

¼ teaspoon ground black pepper

⅛ teaspoon salt

- Put all ingredients in a blender and blend until well combined.
Makes 6 servings of 2 tablespoons each.

Nutrition Information per Serving	
Calories	110.08
Protein	0.10 g
Carbs	0.52 g
Fat	12.52 g
Fiber	0.03 g
Net carb	0.49 g

Red Wine Vinaigrette

⅔ cup extra virgin olive oil

3 tablespoons red wine vinegar

1 tablespoon lemon juice

1 teaspoon Dijon mustard

1 packet Splenda

¼ teaspoon ground black pepper

⅛ teaspoon salt

- Blend all ingredients in a blender.

Makes enough for 4 servings.

Thanks to Robin Hartzell for the recipe for the dressing; she adapted it from her favorite.

Nutrition Information per Serving

Calories	168.21
Protein	0.13 g
Carbs	1.33 g
Fat	18.80 g
Fiber	0.06 g
Net carb	1.27 g

Soy Ginger Dressing

¼ cup rice vinegar

3 tablespoons soy sauce

2 teaspoons grated fresh ginger

2 teaspoons toasted sesame oil

1 packet Splenda

• Place all ingredients in a small jar with a tight lid and shake vigorously. Be sure that the ginger is finely grated. Alternatively, blend in a blender to ensure that all ingredients are well blended.
Makes enough for 4 servings.

Nutrition Information per Serving	
Calories	34.85
Protein	0.77 g
Carbs	1.58 g
Fat	2.34 g
Fiber	0.02 g
Net carb	1.56 g

VEGETABLES

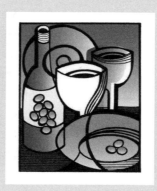

Asparagus in Foil

1 pound fresh asparagus
2 tablespoons lemon juice
4 tablespoons extra virgin olive oil
1 clove garlic, minced
1 tablespoon chopped fresh parsley
salt & pepper, to taste

- Wash and pat dry the asparagus spears. Place in a shallow dish.
- Whisk together the olive oil, lemon juice, minced garlic, parsley, and salt & pepper. Pour over asparagus and marinate for an hour, turning occasionally.
- Place asparagus in the center of a large piece of tin foil and tent, being sure to seal all the seams.
- Place on a BBQ that has been preheated to a medium-high temperature. Cook for 10 minutes. Carefully open the foil wrap to let steam escape.
Makes 4 servings.

VARIATION: Place the foil bag on a cookie sheet and cook in an oven at 400° for 10 minutes.

Nutrition Information per Serving

Calories	149.14
Protein	2.69 g
Carbs	5.95 g
Fat	14.26 g
Fiber	2.46 g
Net carb	3.49 g

Cranberry Salsa

2 large tangerines
3 cups raw cranberries
½ cup pecan halves
12 packets Splenda

• Place the first tangerine, complete with rind, in a food processor or blender and pulse a couple of times. Add the cranberries, Splenda, and nuts. Peel the second tangerine and add it to the food processor. Process until blended but not puréed.

Makes 16 servings of approximately 2 tablespoons each.

NOTE: This is a great garnish with many dishes but especially served with chicken or white fish.

Thanks to my dad, Greg Tompkins, for this simple and tasty idea.

Nutrition Information per Serving	
Calories	41.05
Protein	0.46 g
Carbs	5.01 g
Fat	2.49 g
Fiber	1.43 g
Net carb	3.58 g

Creamed Spinach

10 cups raw spinach
2 tablespoons butter
1 teaspoon cornstarch
¼ cup heavy cream
¼ cup light cream
½ teaspoon ground black pepper

• Wash and pat dry the spinach. Place in a large saucepan with just a ¼ cup of water. Bring to a boil, reduce heat, and simmer for 3–4 minutes, turning constantly with a fork to ensure that all the spinach is cooked.
• Remove from the heat. Do not drain. Add butter and stir to melt and distribute evenly.
• Dissolve the cornstarch in the two creams. Add to the spinach and return to the heat. Cook, stirring constantly until the cream sauce has thickened, about 5 minutes.
• Serve in small side dishes.
Makes 4 servings.

Nutrition Information per Serving	
Calories	153.43
Protein	2.94 g
Carbs	4.91 g
Fat	14.44 g
Fiber	2.05 g
Net carb	2.86 g

Creamy Cauliflower with Rosemary

1 cauliflower, approximately 1½ pounds
1 tablespoon butter
1 tablespoon olive oil
3 small green onions, chopped
1 tablespoon fresh rosemary, roughly chopped
½ cup whole milk
½ teaspoon ground black pepper
¼ teaspoon salt
½ teaspoon cornstarch
¼ cup heavy cream
¼ cup shredded white cheddar cheese

- Roughly chop the head of cauliflower into 6–8 sections.
- Heat olive oil and butter in a large saucepan over medium heat. Add the chopped green onion and sauté for 2–3 minutes.
- Add the milk, cauliflower, and chopped rosemary. Bring the milk to a boil and reduce heat. Cover and simmer the cauliflower until done, about 15 minutes.
- Break the cauliflower into bite-sized pieces using a fork. Dissolve the cornstarch in the heavy cream and add to the cauliflower. Stir to distribute evenly and continue to cook for another 3 or 4 minutes, until thickened.
- Serve the cauliflower with a sprinkle of white cheddar cheese on top.

Makes 6 servings.

Nutrition Information per Serving	
Calories	134.33
Protein	4.33 g
Carbs	7.80 g
Fat	10.45 g
Fiber	2.94 g
Net carb	4.86 g

Creamy Garlic Cauliflower

1 medium cauliflower (about 4 cups of florets)
1 medium onion, minced
2 cups chicken bouillon
2 garlic cloves, minced
2 teaspoons butter
¼ cup sour cream
¼ cup heavy cream
1 tablespoon chopped fresh chives or parsley

- Wash cauliflower and cut into small florets.
- Bring chicken bouillon to a boil in a large saucepan and add cauliflower. Simmer until soft, about 15 minutes.
- While cauliflower is simmering, sauté onion and garlic in 1 teaspoon of butter in a small saucepan over medium heat. Cook until soft, about 3–4 minutes.
- Drain cauliflower when soft. Add cauliflower, onion, and garlic as well as sour cream, heavy cream, and an additional teaspoon of butter to a food processor and process until smooth. You may have to process in batches, depending on the size of your processor.
- At this point, the cauliflower may be refriger-ated or frozen until ready to use. If using immediately, reheat gently in original saucepan. Serve sprinkled with chopped chives or parsley. *Makes 6 servings.*

TIP: This is a great substitute for mashed potatoes, and I often serve it with meat loaf, for just this reason.

Nutrition Information per Serving	
Calories	82.05
Protein	1.22 g
Carbs	3.51 g
Fat	7.12 g
Fiber	0.47 g
Net carb	3.04 g

Creamy Zucchini

2 medium zucchini with skin

3 green onions

1 tablespoon butter

2 cloves garlic, minced

½ tablespoon Dijon mustard

1 cup chicken broth

1 teaspoon dried thyme (not ground)

1 teaspoon Fine Herbs

¼ teaspoon salt

½ teaspoon ground black pepper

1 tablespoon cornstarch

¼ cup sour cream

• Grate zucchini (with skin on) using large holes of grater over paper towel. You should have approximately 6 cups. Squeeze the zucchini to remove most of the moisture.

• Thinly slice the green onions.

• Melt butter over medium heat in a large saucepan. Whisk in the mustard and chicken broth, increase heat, and bring to a boil. Boil uncovered, stirring occasionally, until the liquid is reduced by half. This will take about 5 minutes.

• Add zucchini, onions, thyme, Fine Herbs, salt & pepper. Cook, stirring often until tender, about 4 minutes.

• In a small dish, add some liquid from the pot to the cornstarch to dissolve. Add this mixture back into the pot and continue to boil, stirring constantly until the mixture is thickened. This will take an additional 2–3 minutes.

• Remove from heat and stir in the sour cream.
Makes 6 servings.

Nutrition Information per Serving	
Calories	66.71
Protein	1.29 g
Carbs	4.69 g
Fat	4.92 g
Fiber	1.02 g
Net carb	3.67 g

Crowned Cauliflower

1 medium whole cauliflower
1 cup grated cheddar cheese
¼ cup mayonnaise
2 teaspoons Dijon mustard
½ teaspoon cayenne pepper
½ teaspoon salt

• Wash the cauliflower and remove all leaves and the woody stem. Place the cauliflower on a pie plate with a ½" of water. Cover and microwave until cooked. This will take approximately 10–12 minutes.
• While the cauliflower is cooking, turn on the broiler. Then grate the cheese and mix it with the mayonnaise, mustard, cayenne, and salt to make a paste.
• Remove the cauliflower from the microwave and transfer it to a broiling pan. Cover the top and sides of the cauliflower with the cheese topping (crown the cauliflower!). Grill until the cheese melts and starts to brown.
• To serve the crowned cauliflower, cut it into sections. This is a delicious new way to prepare cauliflower.
Makes 6–8 portions depending on the size of the cauliflower.

TIP: Leftover cauliflower can be refrigerated and reheated the next day.

Thanks to Pat Smith of Red Deer, Alberta, for sharing this with us. Pat suggests adding some of the leftover vegetable to eggs for a yummy omelet in the morning.

Nutrition Information per Serving	
Calories	130.98
Protein	4.78 g
Carbs	2.25 g
Fat	11.73 g
Fiber	0.89 g
Net carb	1.36 g

Dijon Cabbage with Pecans

4 cups cabbage, chopped
1 cup roughly grated carrot
½ cup thinly sliced red onion
1 cup chicken boullion
2 tablespoons butter
½ cup pecans, chopped
2 tablespoons Dijon mustard
½ teaspoon paprika
¼ teaspoon salt
½ teaspoon ground black pepper

• Bring broth to a boil in a large saucepan. Add cabbage, carrot, onion, and salt & pepper.
• Toss ingredients to mix well and cook, covered, for about 5 minutes until tender. Stir occasionally.
• Combine butter, Dijon mustard, and pecans. Pour over vegetables and toss again. Sprinkle with paprika.
Makes 6 servings.

Nutrition Information per Serving

Calories	136.42
Protein	2.49 g
Carbs	8.06 g
Fat	11.59 g
Fiber	3.20 g
Net carb	4.86 g

Fine Herbs

....

1 teaspoon dried thyme
1 teaspoon ground savory
1 teaspoon dried oregano
½ teaspoon dried rosemary
¼ teaspoon dried marjoram
¼ teaspoon ground sage
½ teaspoon dried basil
2 teaspoons dried parsley

• Mix all ingredients together well and keep in an airtight container.
Makes 13 servings of 1/2 teaspoon each.

TIP: I prefer to use the whole dried spices in this blend rather than the ground spices. Doing so adds both texture and flavor.

NOTE: I have included this recipe for a French spice blend because manufacturers no longer seem to be making this mix called Fines Herbes. In some cases, the mixture of herbs is changing and does not taste the same. I use this spice a lot, so I have experimented with various options, and this is the blend that I like the best. I have recently found a new spice blend called Herbes de Provence, a French blend with a slightly different flavor that can be used instead of Fines Herbes.

Nutrition Information per Serving	
Calories	2.58
Protein	0.06 g
Carbs	0.30 g
Fat	0.03 g
Fiber	0.14 g
Net carb	0.16 g

Green Beans with Tomato

1 pound green beans
1 tablespoon butter
1 clove garlic, minced
3 small ripe tomatoes, roughly chopped
2 tablespoons chicken broth
1 tablespoon chopped fresh parsley
½ teaspoon freshly ground pepper
¼ teaspoon salt

• Melt butter over medium heat in a large frying pan and add garlic, salt &
pepper, and parsley. Cook for just 1 minute, until fragrant.
• Add the green beans, chopped tomato, and chicken stock and stir well.
Cover and cook, stirring occasionally, until beans are tender. This will take
approximately 10 minutes.
Makes 4 servings.

**Nutrition Information
per Serving**

Calories	74.69
Protein	2.80 g
Carbs	11.13 g
Fat	3.17 g
Fiber	4.52 g
Net carb	6.61 g

Grilled Eggplant

1 medium eggplant
1½–2 tablespoons light olive oil
2 teaspoons lemon juice
1 tablespoon chopped fresh parsley
1 tablespoon freshly ground pepper

- Preheat the BBQ or grill to medium heat.
- Mix the lemon juice, parsley, and pepper with the olive oil.
- Slice the eggplant into slices between ¼″ and ½″ thick. Brush both sides of the eggplant with the olive oil mixture.
- Place the slices on the grill for 2–3 minutes a side, until golden brown grill marks appear and they are cooked through.

Makes 4–6 servings of 2 slices per serving, depending on the size of the eggplant.

NOTE: Nutrition information is calculated based on 4 servings.

Nutrition Information per Serving	
Calories	80.96
Protein	1.43 g
Carbs	8.38 g
Fat	5.50 g
Fiber	3.46 g
Net carb	4.92 g

Puréed Turnip & Carrots

2 cups cubed turnip
1½ cups sliced carrot
1 tablespoon butter
1 packet Splenda
¼ teaspoon cinnamon

• Bring the sliced carrots and cubed turnip to a boil in a large saucepan. Boil until tender, approximately 15 minutes.
• Remove from heat and drain. Place the cooked vegetables in a food processor or blender with the butter, Splenda, and cinnamon. Process to the desired smoothness. Add salt & pepper, to taste.
Makes 4 servings.

Nutrition Information per Serving	
Calories	69.68
Protein	1.26 g
Carbs	10.55 g
Fat	3.05 g
Fiber	3.18 g
Net carb	7.37 g

Spaghetti Squash with Curried Zucchini

1 spaghetti squash
(approximately 3 pounds)
1 cup grated zucchini
2 tablespoons butter
1 tablespoon curry powder

2 tablespoons sour cream
4 tablespoons heavy cream
2 tablespoons chopped fresh
parsley

• Cut the spaghetti squash in half and scoop out seeds with a large spoon. Place the squash cut side down in a large saucepan and add a couple of inches of water. Bring water to a boil, lower the heat, cover pot, and simmer for 20 minutes.
• While the squash is cooking, prepare the zucchini. Grate zucchini with the skin still on and set aside.
• Melt butter over medium heat in a frying pan. Add the curry powder, 2 tablespoons of water, and the grated zucchini. Sauté over medium heat until cooked, about 10 minutes.
• Put the zucchini mixture, sour cream, and heavy cream in a blender and process until smooth. Add the chopped fresh parsley and blend just a bit. Put back in the saucepan to keep warm while you get the spaghetti squash ready.
• Carefully remove the spaghetti squash from the saucepan and place onto a cutting board. Use an oven mitt to hold the squash while you use a fork to scoop out the meat of the squash. It will form spaghetti-like strings. I like to twirl my fork to make attractive little mounds of the squash on the plates.
• Top the squash with the curried zucchini and serve.

Makes 4–6 servings depending on the size of your squash.

Thanks to my friend Jane Gilmore of Toronto, Ontario, who inspired this recipe.

Nutrition Information per Serving	
Calories	151.12
Protein	1.42 g
Carbs	8.73 g
Fat	13.22 g
Fiber	2.30 g
Net carb	6.43 g

Sweet Tomatoes & Cabbage

2 medium ripe tomatoes
2 packets Splenda
½ cup thinly sliced sweet onion
1 cup sliced cabbage
2 tablespoons extra virgin olive oil
½ teaspoon ground black pepper
¼ teaspoon salt

• Roughly chop tomatoes into ½″ pieces. Sprinkle tomatoes with Splenda and mix in a bowl. Set aside.
• Heat olive oil over medium heat. Sauté the cabbage and onion for 5 minutes, until just soft.
• Add the tomatoes salt & pepper. Continue to cook for an additional 5 minutes. Turn down heat to low, cover the pot, and simmer for a few minutes. *Makes 4 servings.*

Nutrition Information per Serving	
Calories	95.48
Protein	1.25 g
Carbs	7.88 g
Fat	7.36 g
Fiber	1.41 g
Net carb	6.47 g

Zucchini Ribbons

2 medium zucchini
½ medium onion, thinly sliced
1 cup cherry or grape tomatoes
1½ tablespoons olive oil
¼ teaspoon dried thyme leaves
½ teaspoon freshly ground pepper

- Using a vegetable peeler, slice zucchini into long ribbons.
- Heat olive oil in a large frying pan on medium heat. Add onions and zucchini, sprinkle with thyme and pepper, and sauté for 5 minutes, stirring constantly. Add the tomatoes and continue to cook for another 2–3 minutes. *Makes 4 servings.*

Thanks to my friend Dixie Trenholm of Carp, Ontario, who inspired this dish.

Nutrition Information per Serving	
Calories	74.49
Protein	1.67 g
Carbs	6.21 g
Fat	5.54 g
Fiber	1.83 g
Net carb	4.38 g

POULTRY & FISH

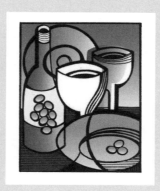

Baked Balsamic Chicken

4 boneless, skinless chicken breasts

3 tablespoons balsamic vinegar

2 tablespoons olive oil

2 cloves garlic, finely minced

freshly ground pepper, to taste

- Preheat over to 375°.
- Combine vinegar, oil, garlic, and pepper to make marinade. Pour over chicken breasts in a shallow bowl, toss to coat, and marinate for 30–45 minutes.
- Spray baking pan with a nonstick agent. Bake the chicken for 40–45 minutes, until done through.

Makes 4 servings.

Nutrition Information per Serving

Calories	209.19
Protein	29.20 g
Carbs	1.25 g
Fat	8.51 g
Fiber	0.13 g
Net carb	1.12 g

Baked Halibut with Sour Cream

1½ pounds halibut fillet
½ cup chopped green onion
1 cup sour cream
¼ teaspoon ground black pepper
¼ teaspoon dried dill
⅓ cup grated Parmesan cheese

- Preheat oven to 350°.
- Place the halibut in the bottom of a well-buttered baking dish.
- Combine all ingredients except the cheese. Pour this thick, creamy mixture over the halibut.
- Bake for 20–25 minutes, depending on the thickness of your fillet.
- Sprinkle with the finely grated cheese and put under the hot broiler just long enough to brown the cheese.

Makes 6 servings.

Thanks to Valerie Caspersen of Victoria, British Columbia, for this great recipe.

Nutrition Information per Serving

Calories	187.22
Protein	17.86 g
Carbs	3.53 g
Fat	11.11 g
Fiber	0.23 g
Net carb	3.30 g

BBQ'd Salmon with Basil Sauce

1–1½ pounds salmon fillets
4 sprigs fresh dill
8 fresh chives
2 tablespoons white wine
1 teaspoon butter
Basil Sauce (see recipe)

• Grease a large piece of tinfoil with butter. Make sure that you have sufficient tinfoil to tent the salmon fillets. Cut the fillets into four pieces.
• Place the salmon on the tinfoil, skin side down. Place two fresh chives and a sprig of fresh dill on each fillet. Sprinkle with a little freshly ground pepper & salt. Pour the white wine over the fish and fold the tinfoil to make an airtight tent over the salmon.
• Place on a hot BBQ for 12–15 minutes, depending on the thickness of the fillets.
• To serve, pour a couple of tablespoons of sauce over the salmon.
Makes 4 servings.

NOTE: Although there is some saturated fat in the mayonnaise in the sauce, most of the fat in this delicious recipe is from the salmon and is the type of good fat that you want to increase in your diet.

Nutrition Information per Serving

Calories	511.74
Protein	22.99 g
Carbs	3.23 g
Fat	44.35 g
Fiber	0.51 g
Net carb	2.72 g

Chicken Cacciatore

3–4 pounds cut-up chicken

½ teaspoon salt

½ teaspoon black pepper

1–2 tablespoons olive oil

1 medium red onion, minced

2 garlic cloves, minced

4 cups sliced fresh mushrooms

1 large can (28 ounces) diced tomatoes

3–4 tablespoons tomato paste

1 cup chicken broth

1 teaspoon dried oregano (not ground but leaves)

1 teaspoon dried basil

½ teaspoon cayenne pepper

2 bay leaves

¼ cup red wine

8–10 cups cooked spinach

• Cut the chicken into reasonable-sized portions. Trim all visible fat and skin. You may use all thighs or all breasts if you wish or buy a whole cut-up chicken.
• Sprinkle chicken with salt and black pepper and brown in hot olive oil over medium heat in a large nonstick skillet or ovenproof stew pot. This may have to be done in batches. Remove chicken from pot and set aside.
• Add onion, garlic, mushrooms, and green pepper to the pot and sauté for approximately 5 minutes or until soft. You may need to add the second table-spoon of olive oil at this point.

continued

- Stir in the chicken broth, being sure to loosen any brown spots at the bottom of the pot. Add the diced tomatoes and tomato paste, stirring to blend. Add the spices and bay leaves.
- Return chicken to the pot. The tomato sauce should almost completely cover the chicken. Place in a 350° oven for 1 hour or until the chicken is tender.
- Remove the pot from the oven and add red wine. If the sauce is a little thin, you may add an additional tablespoon of tomato paste at this point. Return to oven for an additional 30–40 minutes.
- Serve over a bed of steamed spinach.

This dish serves 8.

NOTE: This is a somewhat spicy version of the traditional Italian dish. It freezes well or keeps in the fridge overnight for lunch or dinner the following day.

Nutrition Information per Serving

Calories	555.10
Protein	47.19 g
Carbs	16.51 g
Fat	34.36 g
Fiber	7.69 g
Net carb	8.82 g

Chicken Wrap

4 cabbage leaves
1 cup cooked chicken pieces
   (cubed or thinly sliced)
½ red onion, thinly sliced
½ red pepper, thinly sliced
½ green pepper, thinly sliced
1 tablespoon olive oil

1 tomato, seeded and finely
   minced
½ teaspoon salt
½ teaspoon freshly ground
   pepper
½ cup shredded cheddar cheese

- Rinse the cabbage leaves well and cut out the hard core. Place with ½″ water in a microwave dish and set aside.
- Mince the tomato, add the salt & pepper, and place in a small serving dish.
- Grate the cheese and place in small serving dish.
- Place the chicken pieces in another small dish.
- Heat the olive oil and sauté the onion and peppers for approximately 7–10 minutes, until soft. Just before the vegetables are done, place the cabbage leaves in the microwave and cook for 3–4 minutes on high. Put the vegetables in a small serving dish and bring the cabbage leaves and each of the serving dishes to the table.
- To serve, take a single cabbage leaf, line it with chicken, onion, and peppers, add tomato, and sprinkle with grated cheese.
Roll up the leaf, tucking in any stray edges.
Makes 2 servings of two wraps each.

VARIATION: You may substitute cooked beef for the chicken as a variation. You may use lettuce leaves as the wrap and take it with you to the golf course or the office.

Nutrition Information per Serving	
Calories	258.05
Protein	28.25 g
Carbs	12.79 g
Fat	113.23 g
Fiber	3.67 g
Net carb	9.12 g

Crusted Salmon
with Rosemary Sour Cream

1½ pounds salmon fillets

2 packets Splenda

2 tablespoons Dijon mustard

1 tablespoon sesame seeds

1 tablespoon yellow mustard
seeds

1½ tablespoons chopped fresh
rosemary leaves

½ cup sour cream

½ tablespoon chopped fresh
parsley

½ tablespoon chopped fresh dill

1 teaspoon ground ginger

1 tablespoon chopped green
onion

- Preheat oven to 450°.
- Place salmon fillets, skin side down, on a cookie sheet lined with foil and buttered.
- In a small bowl, mix the mustard and Splenda. Add the mustard seeds, sesame seeds, and chopped fresh rosemary to the mustard mixture. Evenly spread this mixture over the salmon fillets.
- Bake until the salmon is pink throughout, about 10–15 minutes, depending on the thickness of the fillets.
- While the salmon is baking, stir together the sour cream, chopped fresh parsley and dill, and ground ginger.
- Using a spatula, lift the salmon carefully from the cookie sheet. Garnish the salmon with a dollop of the rosemary sour cream and a sprinkle of chopped green onions.

Makes 4 servings.

**Nutrition Information
per Serving**

Calories	410.36
Protein	35.74 g
Carbs	6.74 g
Fat	26.12 g
Fiber	1.92 g
Net carb	4.82 g

Poached Salmon with Citrus Sauce

1–1½ pounds fresh salmon fillet
½ cup fresh orange juice
½ teaspoon ground pepper
¼ teaspoon salt
Citrus Sauce (see recipe)

- Preheat oven to 425°.
- Cut salmon into four equal parts. Place skin side down on a large piece of buttered tinfoil in a baking dish. Sprinkle with salt & pepper.
- Pour fresh orange juice over salmon, fold tinfoil to make a tent, and bake for 8–10 minutes, depending on the thickness of the fillets. You may warm the orange juice in the microwave before pouring over the salmon.
- While salmon is baking, prepare the Citrus Sauce.
- Remove the salmon carefully from the foil tent since it will be full of steam. Let the salmon sit for 2–3 minutes. Place on individual plates and divide the sauce among the servings. Pour the sauce over the salmon.

Makes 4 servings.

NOTE: Do not be distressed by the fat content in this dish. The majority of the fat comes from the salmon, which is full of the "good fats."

Thanks to Linda Porter of Delta, British Columbia, for this wonderful dish.

Nutrition Information per Serving

Calories	408.47
Protein	34.12 g
Carbs	4.22 g
Fat	27.54 g
Fiber	0.02 g
Net carb	4.20 g

Quick Chicken Stir-Fry

2 boneless, skinless chicken breasts
2 tablespoons olive oil
2 cups cabbage, thinly sliced
½ sweet onion, minced
1 cup sliced mushrooms
½ cup sliced celery

½ cup chopped asparagus spears
½ medium sweet red pepper,
  chopped
Oriental Stir-Fry Sauce (see recipe)
½ cup commercial BBQ or stir-fry
  sauce with ½ cup water

• Heat olive oil in a nonstick pan. Cut the chicken into 1″ cubes and add to the pan. Brown chicken on all sides.
• Add the onion and mushroom and continue to sauté until soft. Add the chopped vegetables and continue cooking for 2–3 minutes.
• Mix the water and prepared sauce to blend. Add the sauce to the stir-fry and continue cooking for a couple of minutes. Alternatively, you may make the Oriental Stir-Fry Sauce and add it to the stir-fry. Cover the pan and let simmer for 3 or 4 minutes.
• Steam cabbage until it is just done, approximately 5 minutes. Drain the cabbage if necessary and mound in the middle of the plate.
• Heap the chicken stir-fry over the cabbage.
Makes 2 servings.

VARIATION: Delete the chicken and add extra low-carb vegetables to make a vegetarian stir-fry.

NOTE: The nutrition calculation does *not* include the sauce in this recipe due to the wide variation possible. Be careful about the carb count on the prepared sauce that you use. A good sauce, if you have a few extra minutes, is our Oriental Stir-Fry Sauce as noted in the recipe.

Nutrition Information per Serving

Calories	355.11
Protein	33.90 g
Carbs	20.10 g
Fat	16.70 g
Fiber	7.05 g
Net carb	13.05 g

Ricotta Stuffed Chicken Breasts

4 chicken breasts with bone in, skin optional

300 grams ricotta cheese

4 small green onions, chopped

2 cloves garlic, finely chopped

¼ cup chopped fresh cilantro (or flat parsley)

4 fresh rosemary sprigs

4 fresh sage leaves

4 slices bacon

- Preheat oven to 350°.
- In a small bowl, combine the cheese, green onion, garlic, and cilantro. Be sure to blend well.
- Using a sharp knife, cut a slice into the thickest portion of the chicken breast to make an opening. Stuff the opening with the cheese filling. Lay a sprig of rosemary on top of the filling, inside the opening.
- Wrap the chicken breast with a slice of bacon. You can secure the bacon with a toothpick, if necessary. Lay a fresh sage leaf on top of the chicken breast and under the bacon.
- Bake for 40–45 minutes or until the internal temperature of the chicken breast (not the stuffing) is 170° Fahrenheit. Place the chicken breast under a hot broiler for 2–3 minutes, until the bacon strip is brown and crispy.

Makes 4 servings.

Thanks to Kevin Chenger of Calgary, Alberta, for this great chicken dish.

Nutrition Information Per Serving	
Calories	336.78
Protein	50.16 g
Carbs	3.73 g
Fat	13.28 g
Fiber	0.25 g
Net carb	3.48 g

Shrimp Delight

6 large or jumbo shrimp (raw)
1 tablespoon butter
½ small red onion, thinly sliced
1½ cups sliced fresh mushrooms
1–2 cloves garlic, minced
1 teaspoon freshly ground pepper
1 tablespoon white wine (or sherry)

- Sauté the onion, mushroom, and garlic in butter for about 5 minutes or until nicely soft.
- Add the shrimp and ground pepper and stir until the shells are bright pink.
- Add the white wine (or sherry) just a few minutes before the shrimp are done; then cover and simmer.
- Serve on a lunch plate with a fresh green salad.

Makes 2 servings.

VARIATION: You may substitute olive oil for butter, but the shrimp will not taste quite as rich.

Thanks to Patricia Shaw of North Bay, Ontario, for this great recipe.

Nutrition Information per Serving

Calories	109.58
Protein	6.78 g
Carbs	6.25 g
Fat	6.41 g
Fiber	1.39 g
Net carb	4.86 g

Turkey Stuffing

6 slices low-carb bread
2 cups cabbage cut into 1″
   pieces
1 cup shredded carrot
1 cup chopped celery
1 small sweet onion, minced
1 cup chopped walnuts
½ teaspoon ground sage

1 teaspoon poultry seasoning
1 teaspoon Fine Herbs
½ teaspoon dried oregano leaves
½ teaspoon dried thyme leaves
½ teaspoon parsley
½ teaspoon black pepper
¼ teaspoon salt

• Dry the bread overnight or for 15–20 minutes in a low oven. Break the bread into small cubes. You should have approximately 6 cups.
• Prepare the vegetables and add to the bread crumbs. Sprinkle with spices and mix well with hands to distribute the spices.
• Stuff the turkey cavity and bake as per instructions for the bird.
• This will make enough stuffing for a 10–12-pound turkey.
Makes 20 servings of ½ cup each.

TIP: For additional flavor, and to further reduce the carb content, replace some of the cabbage with chopped pork rinds.

NOTE: The carb content will vary with the bread used. For this recipe, I found and used a sugar-free whole wheat bread that had 11 carbs per slice. Since I developed this recipe, there are now many low-carb breads lower in carb content, and using one of these breads will decrease the total carbs for the stuffing. This dressing stays nice and moist thanks to the vegetables.

Nutrition Information per Serving	
Calories	56.91
Protein	2.10 g
Carbs	5.08 g
Fat	3.83 g
Fiber	1.03 g
Net carb	4.05 g

White Chicken Chili

4 boneless, skinless chicken breasts

4 cups chicken bouillon

1 large sweet onion, roughly chopped

1 large cauliflower

1 garlic clove, minced

2 tablespoons butter

2 celery stalks chopped, with leafy tops separated

2 cups fresh green beans cut into ½" pieces

1 green pepper, chopped

1 teaspoon ground cumin

1 teaspoon cayenne pepper

2 bay leaves

1 teaspoon salt

1 cup chicken broth, if required

2 teaspoons cornstarch dissolved in 4 teaspoons water

chopped fresh parsley, to garnish

- Place the chicken breasts with the water and chicken bouillon in a large Dutch oven or stew pot. Add the leafy tops of the celery ribs and approximately one-third of the chopped onion. Cook over medium-high heat until the chicken is cooked through, approximately 20 minutes.
- Remove the chicken from the pot and reserve the broth. Discard the leafy tops of the celery ribs. Put the cauliflower, cut into small florets, into the broth and cook until soft. This will take 15–20 minutes.

continued

- While the cauliflower is cooking, cut chicken into bite-sized pieces and set aside.
- Melt the butter in a frying pan over medium heat. Add the remaining onion, celery, garlic, and green pepper. Sauté vegetables for approximately 5 minutes, until soft.
- Using an immersion blender, process the cauliflower in the broth. If you do not have an immersion blender, this may be done in a food processor.
- You now have a slightly thickened white sauce. Put in the chicken pieces, sautéed vegetables, green beans, bay leaves, and spices. Stir to blend well. Do not add the chopped parsley until serving.
- Place in a 350° oven for up to 2 hours, until the sauce is further thickened. The liquid should fully cover the chicken and all the vegetables. You may add a little extra chicken broth, if necessary. You may need to add the cornstarch and water 30 minutes before serving, if the sauce has not thickened enough.
- Serve in big bowls and top with shredded cheese, salsa, or sour cream. Garnish with freshly chopped parsley. This dish goes well with a fresh green salad.

Makes 4 servings.

NOTE: This is a great southern twist on the old red chili. It is hot and spicy. You can reduce the cayenne pepper to half, if you find it too hot. The sauce is not as thick as the red variety, but it has a wonderful flavor all its own.

Nutrition Information per Serving

Calories	259.40
Protein	34.60 g
Carbs	18.70 g
Fat	5.88 g
Fiber	7.26 g
Net carb	11.44 g

MEATS

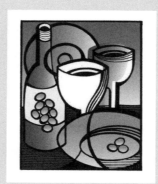

Beef Stroganoff

1½ pounds sirloin steak, ½"–1" thick
½ teaspoon salt
½ teaspoon freshly ground pepper
2 tablespoons olive oil
1 large sweet onion, minced
2 cups fresh mushroom slices
2 cups beef broth
1 tablespoon Dijon mustard
1 tablespoon tomato paste
½ cup red wine
1 tablespoon flour
1 teaspoon cornstarch
2 teaspoons water
¾ cup sour cream
6 cups sliced cabbage
1 tablespoon chopped fresh parsley

• Cut steak into thin slices, approximately 1–2" in length. Sprinkle with salt & pepper.
• Heat the olive oil in a large skillet or stew pot. Add the beef strips and brown on all sides. Add the mushrooms and onion and sauté for 5 minutes or until tender.
• Whisk the mustard and tomato paste into the beef broth until dissolved. Add the broth mixture to the beef and vegetables. Cover, reduce heat, and simmer for 45 minutes.

continued

- Cut the cabbage into long strips about a ¼″ thick. The cabbage will take the place of egg noodles. Bring a large pot of water to a boil just 5 minutes before serving. Put the cabbage in the pot and cook for 3–5 minutes. You want the cabbage to be a little firm.
- While the cabbage is cooking, whisk the flour and cornstarch into the wine with water and add to the beef mixture. Add the sour cream and stir to blend. Cook, stirring constantly, until the sauce is thickened.
- Drain the cabbage well. Serve the beef over the hot cabbage and garnish with chopped fresh parsley.

Makes 6 servings.

TIP: This dish, served over a slice of low-carb toast, is delicious the next day for lunch.

Nutrition Information per Serving

Calories	340.28
Protein	24.29 g
Carbs	16.52 g
Fat	18.96 g
Fiber	6.82 g
Net carb	9.70 g

Braised Pork Loin Chops

6 pork chops, center loin
1 small onion, cut in half and thinly sliced
1 tablespoon olive oil
1 tablespoon chopped fresh rosemary
½ teaspoon ground black pepper
¼ teaspoon salt
½ cup sour cream
⅓ cup heavy cream
2 cups sliced mushrooms

- Preheat oven to 350°.
- Trim all visible fat from the chops. Sprinkle half the rosemary and pepper & salt on the chops.
- Brown both sides of the pork chops in the olive oil. This will take 3–4 minutes a side. Remove to a baking pan.
- Sauté the onions and mushrooms until soft in the same pan used to brown the chops. Add the remaining herbs, sour cream, and heavy cream to the vegetable mixture and stir to blend.
- Pour this mixture over the chops and bake for 30–40 minutes, depending on the thickness of the chops, until tender.
Makes 6 servings.

NOTE: This recipe also works well for boneless pork loin and does not need as much time in the oven without the bone.

Nutrition Information per Serving	
Calories	263.33
Protein	23.63 g
Carbs	2.40 g
Fat	17.51 g
Fiber	0.35 g
Net carb	2.06 g

Cabbage Rolls

1 small head cabbage
11/4 pound lean ground beef
1 cup finely shredded zucchini
1 celery stick, minced
½ cup finely chopped onions
1 egg
2 tablespoons chopped fresh
   parsley
½ teaspoon salt
1 teaspoon freshly ground pepper

Topping
1 medium onion, minced
½ cup chopped celery
½ cup sliced mushrooms
1 garlic clove, minced
2 tablespoons light olive oil
½ cup water
1 can condensed tomato soup
1 tablespoon chopped fresh
   parsley

- Preheat oven to 350°.
- Remove the core from the cabbage and separate the leaves. Microwave the leaves in ½ cup of water for 5 minutes on high and set aside.
- Combine the beef, minced celery, onion, and zucchini in a large mixing bowl. Beat the egg slightly and add it to the beef, along with the chopped parsley and salt & pepper. Mix thoroughly.
- Place approximately ¼ of a cup of the beef mixture in the middle of each cabbage leaf. Roll up, tucking in any edges to make a tight package, and place in a baking dish sprayed with a nonstick agent. Repeat until all beef is used.
- Sauté garlic, remaining onion, celery, and mushrooms in the olive oil over medium heat. Add the tomato soup, water, and chopped parsley.
- Pour the topping over the cabbage rolls, cover, and bake for 1 hour and 15 minutes.
Makes 10 cabbage rolls.

Nutrition Information per Serving	
Calories	220.42
Protein	15.49 g
Carbs	12.15 g
Fat	12.54 g
Fiber	2.55 g
Net carb	9.60 g

Cajun Pepper Steak

1–11/4 pounds sirloin steak, ½"–1" thick
1 teaspoon Cajun or Creole seasoning
1 tablespoon olive oil
1 medium sweet onion, minced
1 medium green pepper, minced
3 garlic cloves, minced
1½ cups beef broth
1½ cups diced canned tomatoes
2 teaspoons balsamic vinegar
½ teaspoon dried basil
½ teaspoon freshly ground pepper
¼ teaspoon salt
6 cups sliced cabbage
1 tablespoon cornstarch
2 tablespoons water

• Cut steak into thin slices, approximately 1–2" in length. Sprinkle with the Cajun or Creole seasoning mix. (This is a blend of peppers and other spices used in southern cuisine. You should be able to find these in the spice section of your grocery store.)
• Heat the olive oil in a large skillet or stew pot. Add the beef strips and brown on all sides. Add the green pepper, garlic, and onion and sauté for 3–5 minutes or until tender.
• Add the beef broth, canned tomatoes, balsamic vinegar, and spices to the beef and vegetables. Cover, reduce heat, and simmer for 45 minutes.

continued

- Cut the cabbage into long strips about a ¼" thick. The cabbage will take the place of mashed potatoes served in the south with this dish. Bring a large pot of water to a boil just 5 minutes before serving. Put the cabbage in the pot and cook for 3–5 minutes. You want the cabbage to be a little firm.
- While the cabbage is cooking, whisk the cornstarch into the water and add to the beef mixture. Cook, stirring constantly, until the sauce is thickened.
- Drain the cabbage well. Serve the beef over the hot cabbage.

Makes 4 servings.

Nutrition Information Per Serving	
Calories	327.13
Protein	33.30 g
Carbs	15.25 g
Fat	14.81 g
Fiber	5.11 g
Net carb	10.14 g

Green Bean Chili

1½ pounds ground round
1 tablespoon olive oil
1 large sweet onion, minced
1 green pepper, minced
28-fluid-ounce can diced tomatoes
10.5-ounce can tomato soup

2 cups green beans, cut into ½" pieces
2–3 tablespoons tomato paste
1 teaspoon cayenne
salt & freshly ground pepper, to taste

- Preheat oven to 350°.
- In a heavy skillet, heat olive oil over medium heat and add the meat. Add salt & pepper to taste and cook, stirring to break up the meat into bite-sized pieces, until completely browned, approximately 5 minutes. Using slotted spoon, remove the meat from the skillet and place in an ovenproof casserole dish or Dutch oven.
- Place onions and green pepper in the skillet and sauté until soft, about 5 minutes. Using the slotted spoon, remove from skillet and add to baking dish.
- Add cayenne, tomatoes, cut-up green beans, tomato paste, and tomato soup and stir until well mixed.
- Place baking dish in the oven and bake for at least 1 hour and up to 3 hours. If baking for a longer period, reduce heat and stir every hour or so to combine and keep from sticking.

Makes 6 servings.

TIP: This chili freezes well and is a bit spicier the next time around.

Thanks to Nancy Shumacher of Lutz, Florida, for the idea of using green beans.

Nutrition Information per Serving	
Calories	325.3
Protein	24.57 g
Carbs	18.42 g
Fat	17.31 g
Fiber	3.62 g
Net carb	14.80 g

Ham & Cheese Roll-Up

1 leaf green lettuce
1 slice ham
1 slice processed cheese
1 tablespoon either mustard or mayonnaise

• Spread the mustard or mayonnaise over the lettuce leaf. Line with the ham and then the cheese slice. Roll up the lettuce leaf, tucking in any stray edges. Wrap in waxed paper and twist the ends to make a secure seal.

NOTE: These make a great little snack and can be carried to work or play (e.g., the golf course). They are also a great breakfast alternative. You can add some cut-up veggies for variety and extra flavor. These are the lowest-carb wraps you can make.

Nutrition Information per Serving

Calories	208.20
Protein	11.54 g
Carbs	1.77 g
Fat	17.25 g
Fiber	0.11 g
Net carb	1.66 g

Oriental Stir-Fry Sauce

3 tablespoons tomato paste
3 tablespoons soy sauce
1 teaspoon toasted sesame oil
2 cloves garlic, minced
1 packet Splenda
2 tablespoons grated fresh ginger
1 teaspoon sesame seeds, to garnish

• Finely grate the fresh ginger. Add the remaining ingredients except the sesame seeds. Whisk all ingredients to blend well.
• Add the sauce to the dish just before finishing. Mix well and continue cooking for 3–4 minutes to ensure that the sauce is hot and well distributed.
• Sprinkle sesame seeds on top of finished dish to garnish.
Makes 4 servings.

NOTE: This sauce may be used as a stir fry sauce for any oriental-style dish.

Thanks to Lisa Shaw of Victoria, British Columbia, for this really simple and delicious sauce.

Nutrition Information per Serving

Calories	31.88
Protein	1.35 g
Carbs	4.32 g
Fat	1.26 g
Fiber	0.60 g
Net carb	3.72 g

Oven-Baked Beef Stew

....

2 pounds trimmed stewing beef
1 tablespoon olive oil
6 carrots
2 cups cubed turnip
6 small onions
6 large celery stalks, including leafy tops
12–18 mushrooms
2 tablespoons flour
1 teaspoon cornstarch
1 teaspoon Fine Herbs
½ teaspoon salt
1 teaspoon ground black pepper

- At least 3½ hours before serving, preheat oven to 350°.
- Trim all visible fat off meat and cut into ½" pieces. Mix together ground pepper, salt, and Fine Herbs. Sprinkle spices on meat and toss to coat.
- Wash all vegetables and cut carrots and turnip into bite-sized pieces. If the onions are very large, cut them into quarters. Put carrots, turnip, and onion into a large bowl of cold water and set aside. Cut the celery into 2" pieces and set aside with the whole mushrooms. Save the leafy tops of the celery.
- In a large stew pot, heat olive oil over medium heat. Brown the meat on all sides. When the meat has been browned, add enough cold water to cover the meat. Scrape any brown bits off the bottom of the pot into the water. Drain and add the carrots, turnip, onion, and leafy celery tops to the pot. Make sure that the water covers the vegetables.

continued

- Cover and bake at 350° for 2 hours, stirring once in a while.
- Remove pot from the oven. Remove any remnants of the leafy celery tops from the stew. (These add great flavor and are often completely incorporated by this time.)
- Turn the oven to 400°. Add the celery sticks and mushrooms to the stew. Make sure that there is sufficient water to cover the vegetables.
- Mix 2 tablespoons of flour with 1 teaspoon of cornstarch in a small bowl. Add hot liquid from the stew a bit at a time to dissolve the flour and cornstarch until you have a very smooth thin liquid. Add this liquid to the stew pot and stir well. This will help the sauce to thicken during the last hour of baking.
- Cover the stew pot and place back in the oven for an hour.
- Serve in large bowls.

Makes 6 servings.

VARIATION: You can add other vegetables to the stew. If you add more delicate vegetables, such as asparagus or green beans, do not add them until the last hour of baking.

Nutrition Information per Serving	
Calories	288.17
Protein	30.07 g
Carbs	20.38 g
Fat	9.69 g
Fiber	5.94 g
Net carb	14.44 g

Pork Stir-Fry

2 tablespoons olive oil
2 cups diced cooked pork
½ cup onion, quartered and thinly sliced
1 cup sliced mushrooms
1 cup diced celery
2 cups chopped bok choy
2 cups zucchini, cut in half and thinly sliced
6 cups cabbage, thinly sliced
Oriental Stir-Fry Sauce (see recipe)

- Heat olive oil in a heavy frying pan over medium heat.
- Add the cubed, cooked pork with the onion and sauté 3–4 minutes.
- Add the zucchini, celery, and bok choy and continue cooking until all vegetables are just done. This will take 4–5 minutes. Stir in Oriental Stir-Fry Sauce and continue cooking for another few minutes until sauce is bubbling.
- While the stir-fry is cooking, steam the sliced cabbage until just done but still firm. This will take 4 or 5 minutes.
- Evenly divide the steamed cabbage on 4 plates. Spoon the stir-fry on top of the cabbage and garnish with sesame seeds.

Makes 4 servings.

NOTE: This is a really tasty way to use up any leftover pork roast or even chops.

Nutrition Information per Serving

Calories	377.85
Protein	24.19 g
Carbs	20.34 g
Fat	24.06 g
Fiber	8.17 g
Net carb	12.17 g

Pot Roast

3–4 pound boneless rump or shoulder roast

3 tablespoons olive oil

1 tablespoon butter

3 sweet onions, cut into 8ths

1 tablespoon paprika

½ teaspoon Fine Herbs

½ teaspoon dried thyme leaves

½ teaspoon dried oregano leaves

3 garlic cloves, crushed

3 leafy celery tops

3 bay leaves

2 cups beef broth

3 tablespoons red wine vinegar (or balsamic vinegar)

½ teaspoon freshly ground pepper

¼ teaspoon salt

6–8 carrots cut into 1½" pieces

1 medium turnip cut into 1½" pieces

1 tablespoon flour

1 teaspoon cornstarch

- Preheat oven to 300°.
- Spray large Dutch oven or covered roasting pan with a nonstick cooking spray. Heat olive oil and butter in the roasting pan over medium-high heat on the stove-top. Salt & pepper the roast and brown on all sides. Remove the roast from pan and set aside.

continued

- Reduce the heat to medium, add the onions to the pan, and sauté for 5 minutes. Add the garlic, Fine Herbs, paprika, oregano, and thyme and continue cooking for 1 minute.
- Add the beef broth and vinegar and bring to a boil. Add the meat back in, then the carrots, turnip, bay leaves, and celery tops. You want to almost, but not completely, cover the vegetables with liquid.
- Cover and place in the oven to cook for 2 hours. After 2 hours, remove the celery tops, turn the roast, and return to the oven for 1 more hour. If there is not sufficient liquid to almost cover the vegetables, add a little extra beef broth. This is not a stew, so it is important to leave some of the vegetables poking out of the liquid so that they caramelize in the oven. At this point, you can add some additional vegetables for variety if desired. Vegetables that blend well with the flavors include mushrooms and asparagus.
- Remove the pan from the oven. Place the meat on a platter and cover with foil. Place the vegetables around the meat for presentation or in a separate serving bowl.
- Mix the tablespoon of flour and teaspoon of cornstarch with a little water in a small dish until they are completely blended and you have a thin liquid. Place the roasting pan on a stove-top element and bring heat to medium. Add the flour and cornstarch and bring the mixture to a boil, stirring constantly until thickened.
- Carve the roast into slices and serve with vegetables and sauce.

Makes 6–8 servings due to shrinkage of the meat.

NOTE: This is a really delicious roast that is moist and full of flavor. It is one of our favorites. It can be kept in the fridge and reheated in a day or two. It also makes a wonderful lunch meal the next day.

NOTE: You can add some squash as a vegetable variation with the other vegetables at the beginning. I might also add mushrooms, green beans, or asparagus during the last hour of baking for additional flavor and color. The carb content will increase slightly with these additional vegetables.

Nutrition Information per Serving	
Calories	391.52
Protein	39.12 g
Carbs	10.41 g
Fat	20.28 g
Fiber	3.01 g
Net carb	7.40 g

Roast Leg of Lamb

3–4 pound leg of lamb
½ tablespoon olive oil
½ teaspoon dried rosemary leaves
¼ teaspoon dried thyme leaves
½ teaspoon ground black pepper
¼ teaspoon salt
2 tablespoons flour
1 teaspoon cornstarch

- Preheat oven to 400°.
- Brush roast with the olive oil. Mix the dried herbs together and sprinkle on the roast. Press herbs into meat with hands.
- Place the roast in a roasting pan and put in the hot oven for 10 minutes to sear the meat and seal in the juices. Turn oven back to 350°. Roast for 45 minutes per pound to allow for the leg bone.
- Remove from oven and let sit for 10 minutes before carving.
- While roast sits, mix the flour and cornstarch into ½ cup of water. Remove all but about a tablespoon of fat from the roasting pan. While stirring constantly, add water mixture to drippings in pan and cook over medium heat until boiling. You may need to add some extra water if the gravy gets too thick. You may also want to add some ground pepper, salt, and Fine Herbs to flavor the gravy.

Makes 6–8 servings, depending on the size of the bone.

NOTE: The nutrition information is calculated using 8 servings.

Nutrition Information per Serving	
Calories	306.82
Protein	35.88 g
Carbs	1.86 g
Fat	16.12 g
Fiber	0.15 g
Net carb	1.71 g

Shepherd's Pie

Creamy Garlic Cauliflower (see recipe)
1½ pounds lean ground beef
½ medium-sized onion, minced
2 cloves garlic, minced
1 teaspoon olive oil
2 tablespoons tomato paste
2 teaspoons Dijon mustard
2 tablespoons water
1 pound green or yellow snap beans
salt & freshly ground pepper, to taste
chopped fresh parsley

- Prepare the Creamy Garlic Cauliflower recipe and set aside.
- Preheat oven to 375°.
- Spray a 3-liter baking dish with a nonstick agent.
- Place the ground beef in a nonstick frying pan, season with freshly ground pepper, and sauté until browned on all sides. This will take 5 or 6 minutes. Break the beef into bite-sized pieces while it is browning.
- Add the onion and garlic to the pan and continue cooking for 3 or 4 minutes, until the onion is soft. Pour or spoon off any fat.
- While the onion is cooking, mix the tomato paste, Dijon mustard, and water in a small dish. Whisk to blend.
- Add the tomato mixture to the beef and continue to cook for 2 minutes while stirring constantly to coat the meat with the sauce. Put the beef into the bottom of the baking dish.

continued

- Wash, trim, and cut the beans into ½″ pieces. Place in water and microwave for 4 minutes. Drain well.
- Place the beans as a layer over the meat. Cover the beans with the Creamy Garlic Cauliflower and sprinkle with some chopped fresh parsley and freshly ground pepper.
- Bake uncovered for 30–40 minutes, until the edges are brown.

Makes 6 servings.

VARIATION: For a slightly sophisticated variation, substitute asparagus spears cut into pieces for the beans. You may also add grated cheese to the topping before baking.

Nutrition Information per Serving

Calories	322.55
Protein	23.52 g
Carbs	7.33 g
Fat	22.22 g
Fiber	1.39 g
Net carb	5.94 g

Sweet & Sour Chops

4 pork loin chops
¾ cup chicken broth
4 packets Splenda
2 tablespoons white wine vinegar
2 cloves garlic, minced
½ teaspoon ground black pepper
1 teaspoon cornstarch

• Heat olive oil in a large frying pan and brown chops on both sides. Cook until almost done, about 4–5 minutes a side. Remove from pan, place in an ovenproof dish, and place in a warm (250°) oven.
• Add chicken stock, Splenda, white wine vinegar, garlic, and pepper to frying pan. Stir to blend well. In a small bowl, add a bit of the liquid to 1 teaspoon of cornstarch to dissolve. Add this liquid to the pan and bring to a boil. Cook, stirring constantly, until thick and bubbly. This will take about 3–5 minutes.
• Return chops to the frying pan, adding any juices from the roasting pan. Turn to coat and stir to blend all juices.
Makes 4 servings.

Nutrition Information per Serving	
Calories	280.17
Protein	18.71 g
Carbs	2.42 g
Fat	21.51 g
Fiber	0.11 g
Net carb	2.31 g

COOKIES

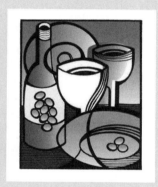

Almond Cookies

2 cups ground almonds
½ cup granular Splenda
¼ cup soy flour
2 teaspoons vanilla extract
½ teaspoon almond extract
2 egg whites
2 tablespoons melted butter

- Preheat oven to 350°.
- Whisk the egg whites until frothy. Add the vanilla and almond extracts and set aside.
- Combine the ground almonds, soy flour, and Splenda in a bowl and mix well. Add the egg white mixture and blend. Slowly add the melted butter, stirring constantly.
- You will have a heavy, sticky dough. Pick up the batter with a teaspoon and use fingers to shape a round, flat cookie about a ¼″ thick. Place on a cookie sheet covered with parchment paper. Repeat until all the batter is used.
- Bake for 20–25 minutes until lightly browned all over.

Makes 3 dozen delicious cookies.

NOTE: If you can't find ground almonds (at the health food store or specialty baking store), you can grind your own using blanched almonds and a food processor or blender.

Nutrition Information per Cookie

Calories	41.34
Protein	1.57 g
Carbs	1.67 g
Fat	3.46 g
Fiber	0.73 g
Net carb	0.94 g

Almond Peanut Butter Cookies

⅓ cup vanilla whey protein

⅓ cup ground almond

½ teaspoon baking soda

8 packets Splenda

⅓ cup soy flour

½ teaspoon baking powder

1 teaspoon xanthan gum

1 cup peanut butter, chunky or smooth

2 eggs

¼ cup olive oil

1 teaspoon vanilla extract

⅓ cup water

- Preheat oven to 350°.
- Mix all dry ingredients in a large bowl and blend well with a wooden spoon.
- Whisk eggs with olive oil in a separate bowl. Add water and vanilla and whisk until blended. Add peanut butter and mix with a fork until completely blended.
- Make a well in the dry ingredients and pour the wet ingredients in the well and stir until fully blended.
- You may either drop by teaspoons or form into small balls and then press with a fork. Place cookies on a cookie sheet lined with parchment paper.
- Bake 10–12 minutes until just brown at the edges.

Makes 4½ dozen cookies.

NOTE: You will want to use commercially ground almonds, sometimes called almond meal, for these cookies so that they blend well. These cookies freeze well and thaw within minutes.

Thanks again to my sister Stephanie, who helped me to develop these really delicious cookies.

Nutrition Information per Cookie	
Calories	49.38
Protein	2.32 g
Carbs	1.27 g
Fat	4.22 g
Fiber	0.10 g
Net carb	1.17 g

Chocolate Coconut Balls

1 can Eagle Brand Milk
5 cups dessicated coconut (unsweetened & fine)
250 grams Lindt 70% Cocoa Dark Chocolate
12 packets Splenda
½ cup butter

• Melt the butter. Mix the coconut and Splenda in a large bowl. Add the butter and milk and blend well. Cover with plastic wrap and place in fridge for 2–3 hours.
• Melt the chocolate in the top of a double boiler, being careful not to let any moisture get into the chocolate.
• Using a small teaspoon, scoop the coconut mixture into your palm and roll into a small ball. Dip the ball into the melted chocolate using a fork or candy dipper. Let drip to allow excess chocolate to come off, and place on a cookie sheet lined with waxed paper.
(I roll about a dozen at a time, then dip them into the chocolate.)
• When the cookie sheet is full, place flat in your freezer for 15–20 minutes.
Makes 100 chocolate balls.

NOTE: I keep my chocolate balls in an air-tight container in the freezer to keep them extra fresh. They take only a minute to thaw.

These are really delicious treats that I make every year at Christmas. The original recipe came from a good friend, Wanda Murphy, of Victoria, British Columbia.

Nutrition Information per Ball

Calories	66.88
Protein	0.76 g
Carbs	4.30 g
Fat	5.22 g
Fiber	0.93 g
Net carb	3.37 g

Crunchy Peanut Butter Cookies

1 cup crunchy peanut butter
½ cup granular Splenda
1 egg

- Preheat oven to 325°.
- Mix all ingredients in a bowl.
- Roll dough into 24 balls. Place balls on cookie sheet covered with parchment paper and flatten with a fork.
- Bake for 12 minutes. Cool before removing from the pan.

Makes 24 cookies.

Thanks to Donna Omeniuk of Winnipeg, Manitoba, for this really great cookie recipe. I think that Donna may have adapted the recipe that appears on the Kraft Peanut Butter jar.

Nutrition Information per Cookie

Calories	71.58
Protein	2.92 g
Carbs	2.54 g
Fat	6.19 g
Fiber	0.00 g
Net carb	2.54 g

Flax Cookies

½ cup butter

12 packets Splenda

1 cup flax seed meal

2 eggs

1 teaspoon vanilla extract

½ cup ground almond

½ cup oat flour

½ cup rolled oats

½ tablespoon baking soda

1 teaspoon xanthan gum

• In a large bowl, cream butter and Splenda with an electric mixer. Add the flax seed meal and blend.

• In a separate bowl, beat the eggs and vanilla. Add the flax seed mixture and beat on low until thoroughly blended.

• Mix all other dry ingredients in a separate bowl.

• Mix the dry and wet ingredients together.

• Separate dough into two equal portions. Form dough into 2 round logs (1" in diameter) and cover with plastic wrap. Place in the freezer to chill for 15–20 minutes.

• Preheat oven to 350°.

• Slice the dough into ¼" thin slices. Place slices on cookie sheet lined with parchment paper.

• Bake for 12–15 minutes, until brown at the edges. Remove to a cookie rack and cool.

Makes 4 dozen cookies.

NOTE: These are really delicious, crunchy cookies that provide great nutrition along with taste.

Nutrition Information per Cookie	
Calories	47.66
Protein	1.45 g
Carbs	2.87 g
Fat	3.97 g
Fiber	1.08 g
Net carb	1.79 g

Icebox Cookies

½ cup oat flour
¼ cup soy flour
¼ cup ground almond
¼ teaspoon baking soda
⅛ teaspoon salt
4 tablespoons butter
⅔ cup granular Splenda
1 teaspoon vanilla extract
1 large egg white

• Combine the flours, ground almonds, baking soda, and salt. Set aside.
• Beat butter at medium speed until light and fluffy, gradually adding Splenda until well blended. Add vanilla and egg white and continue beating until blended.
• Add the flour mixture and stir until combined fully. Turn dough onto a piece of waxed paper and roll into a 6″ log. Put in the freezer for 3 hours or until very firm.
• Preheat oven to 350°.
• Cut the dough log into 24 even slices (approximately ¼″ thick). Place slices 1″ apart on a cooking sheet lined with parchment paper.
• Bake for 8–10 minutes, until the edges and bottoms are just browned. Remove from cookie sheet with a spatula and cool on a wire rack.
Makes 24 cookies.

NOTE: These cookies freeze well and thaw in just minutes.

Nutrition Information per Cookie	
Calories	36.51
Protein	1.04 g
Carbs	2.53 g
Fat	2.84 g
Fiber	0.53 g
Net carb	2.00 g

Maxine's Chocolate Cookies

⅔ cup soy flour

⅓ cup oat flour

⅓ cup ground almond

8 packets Splenda

1 teaspoon baking powder

1 teaspoon baking soda

1 teaspoon xanthan gum

3 squares unsweetened baking chocolate (3 ounces)

2 eggs

¼ cup olive oil

1 teaspoon vanilla extract

¼ cup heavy cream

½ cup finely shredded zucchini with skin

⅓ cup additional ground almond for finishing

- Mix all dry ingredients in a large bowl and blend well.
- Melt chocolate in the top of a double boiler and then set aside to cool slightly.
- Whisk eggs with olive oil. Add cream, vanilla, and zucchini and whisk to blend.
- Make a well in the dry ingredients, add the egg mixture, and mix well. Add the chocolate and stir until all the chocolate is evenly blended. This will make a heavy, wet batter. Cover with plastic wrap and cool in the fridge for 1 or 2 hours. This makes the batter easier to handle.
- Preheat oven to 325°.

continued

Using a teaspoon to pick up the batter, roll into small balls in the palms of your hands. Your hands will get sticky, and you will want to wash and dry between batches. Roll the dough balls into the additional ground almonds, forming a thin layer of ground almond. (You may need to knock off any loose almond meal.) Place the balls approximately 1″ apart on a cookie sheet lined with parchment.

- The cookies will flatten while cooking, and the almond coating will crack to show the dark chocolate inside.
- Bake for 10–12 minutes, until browned at the edges.

Makes 4 dozen cookies.

NOTE: These cookies need to be kept in the fridge because of the zucchini in them. They do not keep for very long. They can also be frozen.

This delicious recipe was given to my mother many years ago by a close friend, Maxine Dennis. My sister Stephanie was instrumental in figuring out the low-carb variety.

Nutrition Information per Cookie

Calories	38.13
Protein	1.59 g
Carbs	1.86 g
Fat	3.19 g
Fiber	0.45 g
Net carb	1.41 g

Oatmeal Peanut Butter Cookies

1 cup crunchy peanut butter
½ cup granular Splenda
¼ cup rolled oats
1 egg

- Preheat oven to 325°.
- Mix all ingredients in a bowl. Roll dough into 24 balls.
- Place balls on cookie sheet covered with parchment paper and flatten with a fork.
- Bake for 12 minutes. Cool before removing from the pan.

Makes 24 cookies.

NOTE: Do not use the instant variety of oats since it will dramatically increase the carb content and the glycemic index.

Thanks to Donna Omeniuk of Winnipeg, Manitoba, for the original idea for these cookies.

Nutrition Information per Cookie

Calories	74.68
Protein	3.05 g
Carbs	3.12 g
Fat	6.25 g
Fiber	0.08 g
Net carb	3.04 g

Oatmeal Raisin Cookies

¼ cup flax seed meal

¼ cup sunflower seeds, finely ground

¼ cup pumpkin seeds, finely ground

½ cup ground almonds

½ cup rolled oats (regular oatmeal, not the instant variety)

½ cup soy flour

6 packets Splenda

1 teaspoon cinnamon

1 teaspoon nutmeg

1 teaspoon xanthan gum

2 eggs

3 tablespoons olive oil

½ cup finely shredded zucchini with skin

¼ cup light cream (half & half)

2 teaspoons vanilla extract

¼ cup seedless raisins

- Preheat oven to 350°.
- Mix all dry ingredients in a large bowl and blend well with a wooden spoon.
- Whisk eggs with olive oil in a separate bowl. Add cream and vanilla and whisk until blended. Add shredded zucchini and mix with a fork until completely blended.
- Make a well in the dry ingredients, pour the wet ingredients into the well, and stir until fully blended.
- Drop by teaspoons onto a cookie sheet lined with parchment paper.
- Bake for 10–12 minutes, until just brown at the edges.

Makes 4½ dozen cookies.

NOTE: These cookies need to be kept in the fridge or frozen.

Thanks again to my sister Stephanie, who did all the preliminary work on these cookies. Can you tell we all have a sweet tooth in my family?

Nutrition Information per Cookie	
Calories	47.17
Protein	2.33 g
Carbs	3.44 g
Fat	3.06 g
Fiber	0.84 g
Net carb	2.60 g

DESSERTS

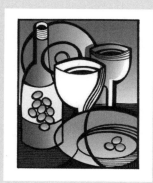

Almond Carrot Cake

1½ cups ground almonds
¾ cup finely grated carrot
1 tablespoon lemon zest
1 teaspoon ground ginger
½ teaspoon ground mace
½ teaspoon cinnamon
5 eggs, separated
11/4 cups granular Splenda
1 tablespoon baking powder
2 tablespoons Grand Marnier
2 tablespoons water
small amount of butter for pan
small amount of granular Splenda
Vanilla Custard Sauce (see recipe)

• Preheat oven to 350°.
• Lightly butter bottom and sides of a 10″ spring-form pan. Sprinkle with small amount of granular Splenda to coat and lightly tap to remove excess.
• In a mixing bowl, combine the spices with the ground almonds and mix well. Add the grated carrots and lemon zest and mix well. Set aside.
• In a deep bowl, beat the egg whites with an electric mixer until they form stiff peaks. (Do *not* use a stainless steel bowl since it will discolor the whites.)
• In a second deep bowl, using the same electric mixer, beat the egg yolks for about 30 seconds. Slowly sift the Splenda into the egg yolks and continue beating for another 3–4 minutes, until the yolks are pale yellow and thick.

continued

- With a wooden spoon, stir the baking powder, Grand Marnier, and water into the egg yolk mixture. Stir well, and this mixture will lighten in texture.
- Add the almond and carrot mixture to the egg mixture, in three equal parts, stirring to blend after each addition.
- Vigorously stir about ¼ of the egg whites into the carrot mixture to lighten it. Spoon the remaining egg whites into the carrot mixture and fold gently with a rubber spatula until no white streaks are left.
- Pour the batter into the prepared pan and bake for 50–60 minutes, until cake tests done with a toothpick.
- Cool on a wire rack for 10 minutes and then remove sides of pan. Cool completely.
- Serve thin wedges of cake with Vanilla Custard Sauce or a little whipped cream.

Makes 10 servings.

Nutrition Information per Serving

Calories	139.84
Protein	6.64 g
Carbs	7.61 g
Fat	9.77 g
Fiber	2.03 g
Net carb	5.58 g

Baked Strawberries & Peaches

4 eggs
9 packets Splenda, divided
1⅓ cups heavy cream
1 teaspoon vanilla extract
2 tablespoons flour
2 peaches thinly sliced
1 cup sliced strawberries
½ teaspoon cinnamon

• Slice the peaches and strawberries and sprinkle with a mixture of 2 packets of Splenda and the cinnamon. Set aside.
• Preheat oven to 325°.
• Place the eggs, 7 packets of Splenda, and vanilla in a large bowl and beat with an electric mixer until frothy. Gradually sift the flour into the egg mixture and whisk to blend thoroughly.
• Pour ¾ of a cup of the egg mixture into a lightly greased 9″ pie plate. Bake for approximately 5 minutes, until the cream is just set.
• Remove the dish from the oven and spread the fruit evenly over the cream base. Pour the remaining cream mixture over the fruit and bake for 25–30 minutes or until completely set.
• Cool for 20 minutes before serving. May be served with a dollop of heavy cream that has been whipped with Splenda.
Makes 6–8 servings.

VARIATION: You may use other berries in place of the strawberries. The carb content will vary slightly.

Nutrition Information per Serving

Calories	201.52
Protein	4.78 g
Carbs	8.08 g
Fat	16.92 g
Fiber	0.99 g
Net carb	7.09 g

Chocolate Almond Torte

4 squares semi-sweet baking chocolate (4 ounces), divided
4 squares bittersweet baking chocolate (4 ounces), divided
1 cup butter, divided
16 packets Splenda, divided
3 eggs
1 cup ground almonds
1 tablespoon orange zest
3 tablespoons heavy cream
toasted slivered almonds, to garnish
small amount of granular Splenda

- Preheat oven to 375°.
- Butter an 8″ round cake pan and line with parchment paper. Butter the parchment paper and sprinkle the sides and bottom of the pan with small amount of granular Splenda. Shake out excess.
- Melt the 2 squares each of the semi-sweet and bittersweet chocolate in the top of a double boiler. Set aside on a tea towel to cool slightly.
- Cream ¾ of a cup of the butter and 12 packets of Splenda (or ½ cup of granular Splenda) together with an electric mixer until fluffy. Add the eggs one at a time, beating well after each addition. With your beater on a low speed, add the chocolate and ground almonds. Stir in the orange zest.
- Pour the batter into the prepared pan. Bake for 20–25 minutes. The center will look soft, and the edges will look done.
- Remove to a cake rack and cool for 20 minutes. Using a small sharp knife, cut around the edges of the pan to release the cake. Invert the pan onto the rack. Peel off the parchment paper, turn cake right side up, and continue to cool for at least an hour.

continued

Glaze
- Melt the remaining chocolate, ¼ cup of butter, and 4 packets of Splenda in the top of a double boiler. Stir to blend while chocolate and butter melt. Cook until fully blended and smooth.
- Remove from heat and beat with a spoon to cool. Add the heavy cream while beating constantly.
- Place waxed paper under edges of cake on serving platter. Pour glaze over cake and allow it to run down the sides. Before glaze has cooled completely, press the toasted slivered almonds into a narrow band on the top of the cake as a decorative border. Gently pull the waxed paper from under the cake. If you like, omit the waxed paper and let the chocolate glaze drip onto the serving platter.

Makes 8 servings.

Nutrition Information per Serving

Calories	412.77
Protein	8.34 g
Carbs	12.80 g
Fat	42.21 g
Fiber	5.85 g
Net carb	6.95 g

Chocolate Mint Cake

Cake
½ cup oat flour
½ cup soy flour
⅓ cup unsweetened cocoa powder
½ teaspoon salt
¼ teaspoon baking soda
¼ teaspoon baking powder
¾ cup butter
12 packets Splenda
2 teaspoons vanilla extract
3 large eggs
½ cup light cream
1 cup miniature semi-sweet chocolate chips

Filling
1 cup semi-sweet chocolate chips
½ cup heavy cream
½ teaspoon peppermint extract

Frosting
6 ounces bittersweet chocolate
½ cup heavy cream
½ teaspoon peppermint extract

Garnish
small red & white mints (or small candy canes, crushed)

continued

Cake
- Preheat oven to 350°.
- Butter 2 round cake pans (8") and line with parchment paper. Butter the paper and up the sides of the pan and dust with oat flour.
- Bring the butter to room temperature. Whisk together the flour, cocoa powder, salt, baking powder, and baking soda until blended.
- With an electric mixer, beat butter until light and fluffy. Add the Splenda, then the vanilla and eggs, one at a time. Add the dry mixture, alternately with the cream, in two batches each, blending well after each addition. Mix in the chocolate chips.
- Pour the batter, evenly divided, into the 2 prepared cake pans. Smooth the batter in the pans until even. Bake in the center of the oven rack until tester inserted in the middle comes out clean. This will take approximately 40–45 minutes, depending on your oven.
- Cool on a cake rack for 5 minutes. Turn cake out onto a cooling rack, peel off the parchment, and cool completely.

Filling
- Place chocolate chips in a medium bowl.
- Bring cream to a simmer in a small saucepan.
- Pour the cream over the chocolate chips. Whisk to melt the chocolate and blend. Continue whisking until smooth. Add the peppermint extract and blend.
- Set aside to cool at room temperature while cakes cool.
- When you are ready to assemble (cakes should be completely cool throughout), beat the filling using the electric mixer until it is fluffy and light in color. This may take a few minutes.
- Place the bottom cake on a flat surface and examine the top to make sure it is flat. If necessary, slice a thin piece off the top to even it out. Spread the filling evenly over the top of this cake and place the second cake on top of the filling and gently press down to make sure that it is secure. Chill for 20 minutes before frosting.

continued

Frosting
- Cut the bittersweet chocolate into small pieces and place in a bowl.
- Bring the cream to a simmer in a small saucepan.
- Pour the cream over the chocolate pieces. Whisk to melt the chocolate and blend. Continue whisking until smooth and shiny. Add the peppermint extract and blend.
- Place the filled cake on a cake rack with waxed paper below the rack. Pour the frosting over the cake and let it run down the sides.

Garnish
- Put a few small red & white mints in the food processor and pulse for a couple of seconds to break them into small pieces. Sprinkle the mint pieces in a border around the top of the cake.
Makes 10 servings.

NOTE: This delicious cake has a high carb count, so I save it for very special occasions and have only a small piece — about half the serving size suggested by the recipe. It presents beautifully with the shiny chocolate frosting and the crushed candies.

Nutrition Information per Serving

Calories	476.26
Protein	8.34 g
Carbs	32.37 g
Fat	38.21 g
Fiber	2.17 g
Net carb	30.20 g

Chocolate Silk Pie

Crust
6 tablespoons butter
½ cup ground pecans
¾ cup ground almonds
6 tablespoons soy flour
¼ cup flax seed meal
1 teaspoon xanthan gum
4 packets Splenda

Filling
3 ounces unsweetened baking chocolate
1½ teaspoons vanilla extract
3 eggs
12 packets Splenda
¾ cup butter

Crust
• Preheat oven to 325°.
• Grind the pecans in a food processor or chop finely with a sharp knife.
• Mix all dry ingredients in a bowl.
• Melt the butter, add to the dry ingredients, and mix well. This will result in a crumble type of batter. Press evenly into a 9″ glass pie plate.
• Bake for 20 minutes, until golden brown.
• Place pie plate on a rack to cool.

continued

Filling
- Melt the chocolate in the top of a double boiler and set aside on a tea towel for a few minutes to cool.
- Cream butter and Splenda with an electric mixer until light and fluffy. With the mixer running at low speed, gradually add the chocolate and vanilla. Add the eggs one at a time, beating on medium speed for 5 minutes after each addition.
- Pour the filling into cooled pie crust and put in the fridge for 2–3 hours.
- Garnish with a small dollop of whipped cream or some fresh berries or a drizzle of chocolate sauce.

Makes 8 servings.

NOTE: This is a real indulgence because of the fat content — creamy, smooth, delicious, and worth the splurge!

Nutrition Information per Serving

Calories	458.97
Protein	9.51 g
Carbs	11.61 g
Fat	42.82 g
Fiber	3.80 g
Net carb	7.81 g

Cooked Raspberry Purée

1 cup raspberries, either fresh or frozen
6 packets Splenda
1 tablespoon liqueur or sweet dessert wine

• Wash and pat dry raspberries if using fresh fruit. Purée the raspberries in a blender or food processor. You may put them through a sieve if you do not want the seeds in the purée.
• Put the raspberries, Splenda, and liqueur in a small pot and cook over medium heat for 5–10 minutes.
• Cool fully before using as a garnish on any one of many cakes or as an ice-cream topping.
Makes 8 servings of 2 tablespoons each.

NOTE: Nutrition will vary slightly depending on your choice of liqueur.

Nutrition Information per Serving

Calories	12.09
Protein	0.09 g
Carbs	3.12 g
Fat	0.00 g
Fiber	0.33 g
Net carb	2.79 g

Flourless Chocolate Cake

6 ounces bittersweet chocolate

2 ounces unsweetened chocolate

¼ pound butter

5 large eggs, separated

⅔ cup granular Splenda

- Preheat oven to 325°.
- Lightly grease an 8″ round pan and line the bottom with parchment paper.
- Melt chocolate and butter in the top of a double boiler, stirring occasionally. Allow to cool slightly.
- Whisk together the egg yolks and all but 3 tablespoons of the Splenda until you have a thick pale yellow mixture. Slowly add the cooled chocolate to the yolks.
- Beat the egg whites into stiff peaks, adding the remaining 3 tablespoons of Splenda as you beat them.
- Stir the chocolate mixture into the egg whites. Pour into the prepared pan and knock gently on the countertop to settle the air bubbles.
- Bake for 40–45 minutes or until toothpick comes out clean. Let cool on a wire rack for 5 minutes and then loosen cake around the edges and invert on a plate. Remove parchment covering, invert again on the rack, and let cool completely. *Cut into 8 wedges.*

PRESENTATION: You will find that this is a very rich cake. I like to serve it with a little whipped cream and a few fresh berries to help provide balance. I particularly like raspberries and blackberries. You could also serve on a berry purée or with a simple Chocolate Ganache (see recipe).

Thanks to Lynne Wilson of Lantzville, British Columbia, for this flourless cake.

Nutrition Information per Serving

Calories	300.39
Protein	6.56 g
Carbs	16.57 g
Fat	25.94 g
Fiber	2.71 g
Net carb	13.86 g

Julie's Middle Eastern Orange Cake

2 large oranges

6 eggs

1 cup granular Splenda

1½ cups ground almonds

1 teaspoon baking powder

• Wash and then simmer the whole oranges in water for 2 hours. Let cool. Quarter and remove any seeds. Place the sections (skins included) in a food processor or blender and process.
• Preheat oven to 375°.
• Line a 9″ spring-form pan with parchment paper.
• If you have a food processor, add all the remaining ingredients to the oranges and mix thoroughly. If you are using a blender, blend the oranges and eggs together, add them to the dry ingredients, and then mix well.
• Pour the batter into the prepared pan. Tap the pan gently on the countertop to even the batter.
• Bake for 50–60 minutes until the top of the cake is lightly browned. This cake does not rise, so it is fairly flat in the pan.
• Place on a wire rack to cool. Unmold the sides of the pan immediately and let cake cool for 10–15 minutes before taking the bottom part off. Cool completely before peeling the parchment paper off the cake.
• Serve with a drizzle of chocolate sauce or some fresh berries and whipped cream.

Makes 10 thin wedges.

NOTE: I have made this cake using 4 small tangerines in place of the oranges, and it was wonderful.

Thanks to Lynne Wilson of Lantzville, British Columbia, for this unusual and yummy cake.

Nutrition Information per Serving	
Calories	143.18
Protein	7.48 g
Carbs	8.99 g
Fat	10.25 g
Fiber	2.31 g
Net carb	6.68 g

Lemon Cream Pie

Crust
¾ cup flax seed meal
¾ cup ground almonds
4 tablespoons butter
5 packets Splenda
1 teaspoon xanthan gum

Filling
1 cup granulated Splenda, divided
4 eggs
½ cup fresh lemon juice (2–3 lemons)
1 cup heavy cream, divided

Crust
•   Melt the butter. Mix the flax seed meal, ground almonds, xanthan gum, Splenda, and butter with a fork to blend well. This will make a sticky crumb mixture. Press into the bottom and up the sides of a 9″ glass pie plate.
•   Bake at 375° for 10–12 minutes, until the edges are brown. Let cool completely.

Filling
•   Take 2 teaspoons of zest from one of the lemons, wrap in plastic, and put in the fridge for use later. Squeeze ½ cup of fresh lemon juice.
•   Whisk the eggs in a large bowl until fluffy. Gradually add ¾ cup of loose Splenda to the eggs. Whisk in the lemon juice and then gradually add ½ cup of the heavy cream.

continued

- Pour this lemon cream mixture into the pie plate and bake at 375° for 25–30 minutes or until the middle of the filling is set. Cool completely.
- To serve, whip the remaining heavy cream with the remaining Splenda and add the lemon rind to the whipped cream. Serve small wedges of pie with the lemon whipped cream on top.

Makes 8 servings.

Nutrition Information per Serving	
Calories	299.79
Protein	8.37 g
Carbs	10.41 g
Fat	29.02 g
Fiber	4.11 g
Net carb	6.30 g

Lemon Custard Cake

2 large lemons

¼ cup flour

½ cup granular Splenda

3 eggs, separated

6 packets Splenda

1 cup whole milk

⅞ cup heavy cream

- Preheat oven to 350°.
- Finely grate the zest of 1 lemon, approximately 1 tablespoon. Squeeze 6 tablespoons of lemon juice from the lemons.
- Whisk together the flour, salt, and ½ cup of granular Splenda.
- Whisk together the yolks, milk, cream, lemon juice, and zest. Add to the flour mixture and stir until just combined.
- Beat the egg whites in a separate bowl until soft peaks form. Add 6 packets of Splenda, 2 at a time, until stiff peaks form and the egg whites are glossy.
- Whisk about ⅓ of the egg white mixture into the batter to lighten. Fold in the remaining egg white with a rubber spatula.
- Pour into a buttered 1½-quart shallow ceramic baking dish. Place this dish inside a roasting pan that has 1–2″ of water in the bottom. Bake until the cake is puffed and golden brown, about 40–50 minutes.
- Cool on a rack for a few minutes and serve warm. This great little cake may also be refrigerated and served again the following day.

Makes 6 servings.

Nutrition Information per Serving	
Calories	137.50
Protein	5.88 g
Carbs	12.27 g
Fat	8.93 g
Fiber	0.92 g
Net carb	11.35 g

Peach Cobbler

3 medium peaches (2½" diameter)

7 packets Splenda, divided

½ teaspoon ground cinnamon

⅛ teaspoon ground nutmeg

¾ cup almond slivers, roughly ground

⅓ cup oats

3 tablespoons butter

1 teaspoon xanthan gum

- Preheat oven to 375°.
- Cut butter into small pieces and let reach room temperature.
- Peel peaches and cut into bite-sized pieces. Mix peaches with 4 packets of Splenda and the cinnamon and nutmeg. Set aside for a few minutes.
- Mix the ground almonds, oats, butter, xanthan gum, and remaining 3 packets of Splenda. This will make a dry, crumbly topping. (I like to leave some of the almond pieces a little bigger to provide more crunch to the topping.)
- Lightly grease a 1½-quart ovenproof casserole dish. Pour peaches into the casserole and top with the oat mixture. Be sure to spread topping evenly and to the edges of the dish.
- Bake for 25 minutes, until the topping is browned and the fruit is bubbling. Let cool for 15 minutes.

Makes 6 servings.

NOTE: May be served with a small dollop of whipped cream or some light or low-carb vanilla ice cream.

Nutrition Information per Serving

Calories	179.74
Protein	4.40 g
Carbs	14.87 g
Fat	12.44 g
Fiber	3.41 g
Net carb	11.46 g

Peaches with Sweet Pecans

1 cup pecan halves
3 tablespoons butter
12 packets Splenda, divided
6 medium peaches (2½" diameter)
½ cup heavy cream
¾ teaspoon cinnamon, divided

- Preheat oven to 375°.
- Melt 1 tablespoon of butter and mix with 4 packets of Splenda and ½ teaspoon of cinnamon.
- Line a baking pan with parchment paper. In a small bowl, toss pecans with the butter and spice mixture. Bake for 5 minutes, stir to turn nuts, and continue baking for another 10 minutes.
- Pour nuts onto a clean chopping board, let cool slightly, and chop roughly.
- Line pan with new parchment paper. Place peach halves in the pan. Melt the remaining tablespoon of butter and add 6 packets of Splenda and ¼ teaspoon of cinnamon. Brush the peach halves with this mixture and bake for 25–30 minutes until nicely browned on top.
- Place two peach halves on a dessert plate, sprinkle with roasted nuts, and top with a dollop of heavy cream whipped with 2 packets of Splenda.

Makes 6 servings, or serve 12 half peaches with the nuts and cream.

Nutrition Information per Serving	
Calories	286.09
Protein	2.80 g
Carbs	15.98 g
Fat	26.14 g
Fiber	3.73 g
Net carb	12.25 g

Pumpkin Custard

1½ cups heavy cream

12 packets Splenda

½ teaspoon rum extract

4 large egg yolks

1 cup canned pumpkin (not pie filling)

½ teaspoon cinnamon

¼ teaspoon nutmeg

¼ teaspoon ground cloves

⅛ teaspoon ground mace

⅛ teaspoon ground ginger

- Preheat oven to 325°.
- In a large saucepan, whisk together the cream, rum extract, spices, and Splenda. Heat over medium heat until steam rises and bubbles form around the edges. Remove from heat, whisking every minute or so to keep blended.
- In a large bowl, whisk the egg yolks until light and fluffy. Add pumpkin and whisk to blend. Very slowly add the warm cream mixture to the egg mixture until well blended.
- Pour into 6 small ramekins or individual custard cups. Fill a large roasting pan with ½" of water and place the 6 dessert dishes in the water bath. Put the roasting pan in the oven and bake for 30–40 minutes, until just set. The mixture will appear slightly soft in the middle.
- Carefully remove ramekins from roasting pan, making sure not to get any water in the custards, and place on a wire rack to cool. Place in the fridge for 2–3 hours before serving. Serve with a small dollop of whipped cream.

Makes 6 servings.

NOTE: This is like a Créme Brûlée with a pumpkin flavoring. It is delicious.

Nutrition Information per Serving	
Calories	268.02
Protein	3.75 g
Carbs	27.28 g
Fat	25.46 g
Fiber	20.01 g
Net carb	27.27 g

Raspberries & Cream

1½ cups fresh or frozen raspberries
¾ cup heavy cream
2 packets Splenda
2 slices (¼") pound cake

Raspberry Sauce
juice of berries
2 teaspoons liqueur
¼ teaspoon xanthan gum

- This recipe works best with frozen, unsweetened raspberries. If you are using fresh raspberries, you will want to mash a few to make the purée.
- Thaw the berries and strain. Put berries in the fridge until needed. Take the liquid and place in a small saucepan. Add the liqueur (a fruit flavor works best) and the xanthan gum and whisk ingredients together. Turn the heat to medium and continue whisking while it cooks for 2–3 minutes. The sauce will thicken (due to the liqueur and the xanthan gum) as it cooks.
- Remove from heat and let cool. It will continue to thicken as it cools. If your sauce gets too thick to pour, you can thin it a bit with water.
- Whip the heavy cream with the Splenda until fairly stiff.
- Cut the two slices of pound cake into small cubes.
- Assemble just an hour before serving, or the whipped cream breaks down. Keep in the fridge until ready to serve. You can assemble in four glass dessert dishes, but I particularly like the appearance when it is assembled in a martini glass.

continued

- Evenly divide the cake cubes among the four dishes and place them in the bottom. They do not need to be even or flat. Pour the raspberry sauce over the cake and let it run down the sides of the dish. Spoon a little of the whipped cream over the drenched cake. Divide the berries evenly among the dishes, reserving one raspberry as garnish for each dish. Spoon the remaining whipped cream over the berries, reaching to the edge of the dish if possible. Place a single berry on top of each dish.
- This is a delicious dessert that is beautiful to look at due to the layered effect of the berries and cream.

Makes 4 servings.

NOTE: I usually don't use all the raspberry sauce when I assemble this dessert. Any extra sauce can be served over low-carb ice cream or any other small treat the following day.

Nutrition Information per Serving	
Calories	182.24
Protein	1.53 g
Carbs	13.17 g
Fat	14.26 g
Fiber	3.14 g
Net carb	10.03 g

Raspberry Cheesecake

Crust

1 cup pecan pieces (or walnut)

1 cup almond pieces

2 packets Splenda

1 teaspoon xanthan gum

2 tablespoons melted butter

Filling

2 packages (250 grams each) light cream cheese

2 packages (250 grams each) cream cheese

4 large eggs

¼ cup heavy cream

2 teaspoons vanilla extract

10 packets Splenda

Topping

2 cups fresh (or frozen, unsweetened) raspberries

4 packets Splenda

4 teaspoons lemon juice

- Preheat oven to 325°.
- Butter a 9″ spring-form pan and set aside.
- Finely chop the nuts or put in a food processor and pulse for about 10 seconds. You do not want the nuts to be powdered but finely chopped. Add the melted butter, xanthan gum, nuts, and Splenda and mix well. Press the crust into the pan and bake for 10–12 minutes or until lightly browned. Remove from the oven and let cool.

continued

- Allow the cream cheese to come to room temperature and beat with an electric mixer until smooth. This is easier to do if you chop the cream cheese into pieces before beating. Add the Splenda and continue beating. Add the eggs one at a time and beat the mixture after each egg. Add the heavy cream and vanilla extract and beat well to mix all ingredients.
- Pour the cheese mixture into the spring-form pan and even out the top with a spatula.
- Put the raspberries, lemon juice, and Splenda into a blender or food processor and purée. (If using frozen berries, they must be completely thawed before blending.) You may strain the purée if you don't like the seeds.
- Using approximately ¼ of the raspberry purée, drop it by spoonfuls on top of the cheese mixture, distributing the spoonfuls around the perimeter of the pan. Using a sharp knife, "cut" into the raspberry purée dollops and drag out to points. Do this 2 or 3 times for each dollop of raspberry, making an attractive pattern on top of the cake.
- Place the pan in the middle of the oven and bake for 55–60 minutes, until set and slightly brown at the edges. Remove from the oven and place on a cookie rack to cool.
- After about 10 minutes, take a sharp knife and run the blade around the perimeter before loosening the sides of the pan. Let the cheesecake cool completely and then place it in the fridge until serving time. I do not try to take the cake off the bottom of the spring form. If I want to take the cheesecake to the table to serve, I just place the spring-form bottom on an attractive serving plate.
- To serve, place a piece of cheesecake on a dessert plate and drizzle the plate with the remaining raspberry purée. This is easiest to do with a small squeeze bottle sold in kitchen and dollar stores.

Makes 10–12 servings.

NOTE: This cheesecake presents beautifully for a special occasion with its red raspberry top and garnish. I have had guests tell me that it was the best cheesecake they ever tasted!

Nutrition Information per Serving

Calories	415.49
Protein	11.56 g
Carbs	8.64 g
Fat	39.09 g
Fiber	1.62 g
Net carb	7.02 g

Vanilla Custard Sauce

1 cup milk
½ cup heavy cream
1 long vanilla bean (6")
4 egg yolks
10 packets Splenda
1 teaspoon cornstarch

• Combine milk, cream, and vanilla bean in a heavy saucepan. Place the saucepan over medium heat and bring the liquid just to a boil.
• Remove from heat and let stand for 10 minutes to absorb the vanilla flavor. Stir occasionally while cooling.
• In a mixing bowl, whisk the egg yolks until smooth. Gradually add the Splenda and continue whisking until the mixture is paler yellow and creamy — about 3 minutes. Add in the cornstarch and whisk well to blend. Stir the milk mixture into the yolks, whisking vigorously.
• Return this mixture to the saucepan and cook over low heat, stirring constantly, until the mixture is quite thick and coats the back of a wooden spoon. This will take 10–15 minutes. Do not let the custard boil at this point.
• Remove from heat and let cool, stirring frequently. Remove the vanilla bean, cover the custard, and chill.
• Serve as a sauce to be poured over individual servings of almond carrot cake.
Makes 12 servings of 3 tablespoons each.

NOTE: This is a really delicious vanilla custard sauce. It can be used warm or chilled over fruit or any low-carb cake.

Nutrition Information per Serving

Calories	70.69
Protein	1.80 g
Carbs	2.32 g
Fat	6.05 g
Fiber	0.01 g
Net carb	2.31 g

Warm Chocolate Sauce

⅔ cup and 1½ tablespoons heavy cream
1 tablespoon butter
½ teaspoon vanilla extract
100 grams Lindt 70% Cocoa Dark Chocolate

• Melt butter over medium heat in a small saucepan. Add cream and stir to combine while heating until hot (but not boiling).
• Remove from heat and add roughly chopped chocolate. Stir vigorously until chocolate is melted.
• Add the vanilla.
• For a slightly thinner sauce, increase the amount of cream.
• Use immediately as a sauce over low-carb cakes, low-carb ice cream, or fresh fruit. Or store at room temperature in an airtight container and reheat slowly to use at another time. If the chocolate and butter separate when reheating, use a little extra hot cream to help emulsify.
Makes 8 servings of 2 tablespoons each.

Nutrition Information per Serving	
Calories	126.14
Protein	1.21 g
Carbs	4.45 g
Fat	11.46 g
Fiber	0.63 g
Net carb	3.82 g

Warm Spicy Strawberries

2 cups sliced strawberries
4 packets Splenda, divided
½ teaspoon cinnamon

- Slice the strawberries and sprinkle with a mixture of Splenda and the cinnamon.
- Microwave the fruit for 30 seconds at high power. Stir to blend. Microwave a second time for 20 seconds and stir well. Let the berries sit for approximately 20 minutes. Just before serving, microwave for 10 seconds to reheat.
- Serve warm with a dollop of whipped cream, over some low-carb ice cream, or just as is.

Makes 4 servings.

Nutrition Information per Serving

Calories	27.16
Protein	0.46 g
Carbs	6.50g
Fat	0.28 g
Fiber	1.87 g
Net carb	4.63 g

Warm Strawberries with Peaches

2 peaches, thinly sliced
1 cup sliced strawberries
4 packets Splenda, divided
1 teaspoon cinnamon

- Slice the peaches and strawberries and sprinkle with a mixture of Splenda and cinnamon.
- Microwave the fruit for 30 seconds at high power. Stir to blend. Microwave a second time for 20 seconds and stir well. Let the fruit sit for approximately 20 minutes. Just before serving, microwave for 10 seconds to reheat.
- Serve warm with a dollop of whipped cream, over some low-carb ice cream, or just as is.

Makes 4 servings.

VARIATION: You may use other berries in place of the strawberries. The carb content will vary slightly.

Nutrition Information per Serving

Calories	48.59
Protein	0.81 g
Carbs	11.93 g
Fat	0.32 g
Fiber	2.85 g
Net carb	9.08 g

White & Dark Chocolate Mousse

200 grams Lindt White Chocolate
200 grams Lindt 70% Cocoa Dark Chocolate
2½ cups heavy cream, divided

- Melt the white and dark chocolate separately in tops of double boilers. Set aside on tea towels to cool slightly.
- Divide the heavy cream into two equal portions of 11/4 cups each. In separate bowls, whip the cream just to the soft-peak stage.
- Fold the chocolate separately into each cream mixture using a rubber spatula. You will have a bowl of white chocolate mousse and another bowl of dark chocolate mousse. You may either place each mousse into a separate pasty bag or use a spoon to finish.
- Layer the white and dark mousse into an attractive serving bowl or into martini glasses. Place in the fridge to chill for 2–3 hours. Garnish with a few fresh berries.

Makes 8 servings.

NOTE: This is another indulgence, but it is absolutely gorgeous to look at in clear martini glasses, and it tastes wonderful. Save this dessert for those special occasions.

Thanks to Monique Coyle, who inspired me to develop this dish. She received the original version of this recipe from the chef at the Royal Colwood Golf and Country Club in Victoria, British Columbia.

Nutrition Information per Serving

Calories	537.84
Protein	5.27 g
Carbs	23.95 g
Fat	46.48 g
Fiber	1.25 g
Net carb	22.70 g

CARBOHYDRATE COUNTER

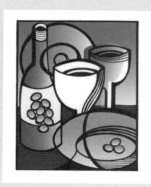

Carbohydrate Counter

The Carbohydrate Counter below provides the number of grams of carbohydrate (in a normal serving) of many common foods. We have included the GI and have calculated the GL where possible. You will note that the GI has not yet been determined for many foods. For those foods you will have to work with the grams of carb provided. Our values for the GI are taken from the 1995 paper by Foster-Powell and Miller. Where a food contains no carbs (pure fat or protein), serving size is irrelevant and therefore appears as —.

Food	Serving size	Carb (gms)	GI	GL
Acorn squash, baked, cubed	1/2 cup	14.9		
Acorn squash, boiled, mashed	1/2 cup	10.7		
Alcohol, distilled (gin, rum, vodka, whiskey)	—	0.0	0	
Alfalfa seeds, sprouted, raw	1 cup	1.3		
Allspice, ground	1 tbsp	4.3		
Almond butter	1 tbsp	3.4		
Almonds, dried	22 kernels	5.8		
Almonds, dry roasted	1 oz	6.9		
Almonds, honey roasted	1 oz	7.9		
Almonds, oil roasted	1 oz	4.5		
Anchovy, fresh or canned in oil	—	0.0	0	
Anise seed	1 tbsp	3.5		
Apple, fresh with peel	2 3/4"	21.1	38	8
Apple, fresh with peel, sliced	1/2 cup	8.4		
Apple, fresh, peeled	2 3/4"	19.0		
Apple, fresh, peeled, sliced	1/2 cup	8.2		
Apple, dried, sulfured, uncooked	2 oz	37.4	29	10

Food	Serving size	Carb (gms)	GI	GL
Apple butter	1 tbsp	8.6		
Apple juice, sweetened	8 fl oz	28.8	60	17
Apple juice, unsweetened	8 fl oz	26.5	41	11
Applesauce, sweetened	1/2 cup	25.5		
Applesauce, unsweetened	1/2 cup	13.8		
Apricots, canned, in juice	1/2 cup	15.3	64	10
Apricots, dried, sulfured	2 oz	35.0	30	11
Apricots, fresh	3 medium	11.8	57	7
Apricots, fresh, pitted, halves	1/2 cup	8.6		
Apricots, with syrup and skin	1/2 cup	27.6	64	18
Apricot nectar	6 fl oz	27.1		
Arrowroot, boiled	1" corm	1.9		
Artichoke, globe, fresh, boiled	1 medium	15.1		
Artichoke hearts, fresh, boiled	1/2 cup	9.4		
Arugula, raw, trimmed	1/2 cup	4.1		
Asparagus, fresh, boiled	4 spears	2.5		
Asparagus, frozen, boiled	4 spears	2.9		
Asparagus, canned with liquid	1/2 cup	2.8		
Avocados, California, raw	1 medium	12.0		
Avocados, California, puréed	1/2 cup	8.0		
Bacon, cooked	2 slices	0.0	0	
Bacon bits, imitation	1 1/2 tbsp	2.0		
Bacon bits, real	1 tbsp	0.0	0	
Bagel, egg	3 1/2" dia	37.6		
Bagel, plain, white	3 1/2" dia	37.9	72	27
Baguette, plain, white	1 medium	15.9	95	15
Baked beans, plain	1/2 cup	26.1	38	10
Baked beans in tomato sauce	1/2 cup	24.4	48	12
Baked beans with franks	1/2 cup	19.7		
Baked beans with pork, sweet sauce	1/2 cup	26.5		

Food	Serving size	Carb (gms)	GI	GL
Baking powder and baking soda	1 tsp	0.0	0	0
Bamboo shoots, fresh, boiled	1/2" slices	1.2		
Bamboo shoots, canned	1/2 cup	2.1		
Bamboo shoots, fresh, raw	1/2´ slices	4.0		
Banana, raw	8 3/4" long	26.7	52	14
Banana chips	1 oz	16.6		
Barbecue sauce	2 tbsp	10.0		
Barley, pearled, cooked	1 cup	44.3	25	11
Basil, dried, crumbled	1 tsp	0.9		
Basil, fresh	6 med lvs	0.2		
Bass	—	0.0	0	
Bay leaf, dried	1 tbsp	0.9		
Bean sprouts, canned	1 cup	1.0		
Bean sprouts, fresh	1 oz	1.9		
Beechnuts, dried	1 oz	9.5		
Beef, any cut	—	0.0	0	
Beef, corned	0.5	0.0	0	
Beef, gravy	1/4 cup	4.0		
Beef, jerky, chopped	1 oz	4.1		
Beef, pie	1 small	12.9	45	6
Beer, lite	12 oz	4.8		
Beer, regular	12 oz	13.2		
Beet, canned	1/2 cup	6.1	64	4
Beet, canned, pickled	1/2 cup	18.5		
Beet, fresh, boiled	1/2 cup	10.0	64	6
Beet greens, boiled	1/2 cup	1.9		
Beet greens, raw	1/2 cup	0.8		
Biscuit, baked	1 oz piece	13.5		
Biscuit, dry mix	2 oz piece	27.6		
Biscuit, plain or buttermilk	1.2 oz piece	17.0		

Food	Serving size	Carb (gms)	GI	GL
Black bean, dried, boiled	1/2 cup	20.4	42	9
Black bean sauce	1 tbsp	2.0		
Blackberries, fresh	1 cup	8.7		
Bloody Mary, from recipe	8 fl oz	7.2		
Blueberries, canned in syrup	1/2 cup	28.2		
Blueberries, dried	1/4 cup	33.2		
Blueberries, fresh	1/2 cup	10.2		
Bluefish	—	0.0	0	
Bologna, beef or pork	1 med slice	0.3		
Bouillon, beef, dehydrated	1 cube	0.6		
Bouillon, chicken, dehydrated	1 cube	1.1		
Bourbon and soda, from recipe	1 fl oz	—		
Boysenberry, fresh	1 cup	18.7		
Bran, see "Cereal" and specific grains				
Bratwurst, pork, cooked	1 oz	1.0		
Brazil nuts, shelled	8 kernels	4.3	0	0
Bread, barley kernel	1 slice	12.8	43	6
Bread, French	1 slice	14.7		
Bread, hamburger bun, white	1 bun	17.7	61	11
Bread, Italian	1 slice	15.0		
Bread, kaiser rolls	1 roll	18.7	73	14
Bread, multigrain, 9 grain	1 slice	13.1	43	6
Bread, oat bran	1 slice	12.0	50	6
Bread, oatmeal	1 slice	13.8		
Bread, pita, white	6 1/2" dia	33.4	57	19
Bread, protein	1 slice	12.4		
Bread, pumpernickel	1 slice	15.0	41	6
Bread, raisin	1 slice	14.8		
Bread, rice bran	1 slice	12.3	72	9
Bread, rye	1 slice	16.0	41	7

Food	Serving size	Carb (gms)	GI	GL
Bread, sourdough	1 slice	13.5	57	7
Bread, white, wheat	1 slice	14.0	71	10
Bread, wheat bran or germ	1 slice	17.0		
Bread, whole wheat	1 slice	13.1	69	9
Bread crumbs, dry, grated	1/4 cup	19.5	71	14
Breadstick	4 oz stick	6.8	71	5
Broad beans, fresh, boiled	4 oz	11.5	79	9
Broad beans, fresh, raw	1/2 cup	6.4		
Broad beans, canned with liquid	1/2 cup	15.9		
Broad beans, dried, boiled	1/2 cup	16.7		
Broccoli, fresh, boiled	1 stalk	3.9		
Broccoli, raw, chopped	1/2 cup	2.0	0	0
Brown gravy, mix, prepared	1/4 cup	3.3		
Brownie	2 oz piece	35.8		
Brussel sprouts, fresh, boiled	1/2 cup	6.9		
Buckwheat	3/4 cup	30	54	16
Butter, any kind	—	0.0	0	
Buttermilk, see "Milk"				
Butternut squash, boiled, mashed	1/2 cup	12.1		
Butternut squash, cubed	1/2 cup	10.7		
Butterscotch topping	2 tbsp	27.0		
Cabbage, boiled, shredded	1/2 cup	3.4		
Cabbage, raw, shredded	1/2 cup	1.9	0	0
Cabbage, Chinese, boiled	1 cup	3.2		
Cabbage, Chinese, raw	1 cup	1.4		
Cabbage, red, boiled, shredded	1 cup	7.2		
Cabbage, red, raw, shredded	1 cup	4.6		
Cake, angel food, 12 oz cake	1/12 cake	29.0	67	18
Cake, banana	1/8 cake	38.0	47	18
Cake, Boston cream, 20 oz cake	1/12 cake	19.8		

Food	Serving size	Carb (gms)	GI	GL
Cake, cheesecake	1 oz piece	7.2		
Cake, chocolate, 18 oz cake	1/12 cake	57.9	38	22
Cake, coffee cheese	1 oz piece	12.8		
Cake, fruitcake	1 oz piece	17.8		
Cake, pound	1 oz piece	24.9	54	13
Cake, sponge, 16 oz cake	1/12 cake	36.6	46	17
Cake mix, angel food, 9" cake	1/12 cake	29.3		
Cake mix, Black Forest, with icing, 9" cake	1/12 cake	55.1		
Cake mix, carrot, with icing, 9" cake	1/12 cake	32.7		
Cake mix, cheesecake, 9" cake	1/12 cake	23.9		
Cake mix, chocolate devil's, 9" cake	1/12 cake	31.8		
Cake mix, gingerbread, 9" cake	1/12 cake	26.3		
Cake mix, white without icing, 9" cake	1/12 cake	34.4	42	14
Candy, 3 Musketeers	2.13 oz bar	46.1		
Candy, After Eight	5 pieces	32.0		
Candy, Baby Ruth	2.1 oz bar	37.2		
Candy, Butterfinger	2.1 oz bar	41.0		
Candy, caramels	1 oz	21.8		
Candy, caramels, chocolate	1 oz	24.7		
Candy, chocolate, milk	1 oz	16.8	49	8
Candy, gum, chewing	1 piece	2.9		
Candy, gumdrops	1 oz	28.0		
Candy, hard candy	1 oz	19.3		
Candy, jellybeans	10 large	24.4	80	20
Candy, Kit Kat	1.5 oz bar	25.8		
Candy, Life Savers, butter rum	4 pieces	20.0	70	14
Candy, M & M's, plain	1 oz	19.3		
Candy, Mars	1.76 oz bar	31.4	68	21
Candy, marshmallows	1 oz	23.0		
Candy, Milky Way	2.15 oz bar	43.7		

Food	Serving size	Carb (gms)	GI	GL
Candy, Mr. Goodbar	2.8 oz bar	40.5		
Candy, Oh Henry!	2 oz bar	36.9		
Candy, peanut brittle	1 oz	19.7		
Candy, peanuts, milk chocolate	1 oz	14.0		
Candy, raisins, milk chocolate	1 oz	19.4		
Candy, Reese's Pieces	1.96 oz pkg	34.1		
Candy, Skittles	2.3 oz pkg	62.4	70	44
Candy, Skor	1.4 oz bar	22.1		
Candy, Snickers	2.16 oz bar	36.8	68	25
Candy, Twizzlers	2.5 oz pkg	65.9		
Cane syrup	1 tbsp	13.4		
Cantaloupe	1/2 x 5" dia	22.3	65	15
Caraway seed	1 tbsp	3.5		
Cardamom, ground	1 tbsp	4.1		
Carrot juice	8 oz	23	43	10
Carrots, baby, fresh, raw	1 large	1.2		
Carrots, fresh, boiled, sliced	1/2 cup	8.2	49	4
Carrots, fresh, raw, shredded	1/2 cup	5.6		
Carrots, frozen, boiled, sliced	1/2 cup	5.8		
Carrots, whole, fresh, raw	7 1/2" long	7.3	47	3
Cashew nuts, dry roasted	14 large	9.3	22	2
Cashew nuts, oil roasted	14 large	8.1		
Cauliflower, boiled	1/2 cup	2.5		
Cauliflower, green, boiled	1/2 cup	3.7		
Cauliflower, green, raw	1/2 cup	3.0		
Cauliflower, raw	1/2 cup	5.0	0	0
Celeriac, boiled	1/2 cup	4.6		
Celeriac, raw	1/2 cup	10.4		
Celery, boiled, diced	1 cup	6.0		
Celery, raw	7 1/2" stock	1.5	0	0

Food	Serving size	Carb (gms)	GI	GL
Celery salt	1 tsp	0.6	0	0
Celery seed	1 tbsp	2.5		
Cereal, All Bran Extra Fiber	1/2 cup	20.0	30	7
Cereal, Bran Buds	1/2 cup	18.4	58	11
Cereal, bran flakes	1 cup	22.0	74	16
Cereal, bran flakes with raisins	1 cup	43.0	75	32
Cereal, Cheerios	1 cup	18.4	74	14
Cereal, corn flakes	1 cup	26.0	80	21
Cereal, Cream of Wheat	1/2 cup	22.5	66	15
Cereal, Cream of Wheat, instant	1/2 cup	22.5	74	17
Cereal, Fruit Loops	1 cup	26.1	69	18
Cereal, granola	1/2 cup	40.0		
Cereal, muesli	1 cup	16	66	11
Cereal, multigrain	1 cup	25.0		
Cereal, oat bran	1 cup	30.0	59	18
Cereal, oatmeal	1/2 cup	22.5	42	9
Cereal, oatmeal, instant	1/2 cup	22.5	65	15
Cereal, oats	1 cup	24.0		
Cereal, puffed rice	1 cup	15.0	82	12
Cereal, puffed wheat	1 cup	21.2	67	14
Cereal, rice	1 cup	35.0		
Cereal, shredded wheat	2 pieces	38.0	67	25
Cereal, Special K	1 cup	20.8	69	14
Chapati, corn, India	1 average	23.3	66	15
Chard, Swiss, boiled, chopped	1 cup	7.0		
Chard, Swiss, raw	1 cup	1.4		
Cheese, blue	1 oz	0.6		
Cheese, brick	1 oz	0.8		
Cheese, brie or camembert	1 oz	0.1	0	0
Cheese, cheddar	1 oz	0.4	0	0

Food	Serving size	Carb (gms)	GI	GL
Cheese, colby	1 oz	0.7		
Cheese, cottage, 1% fat	1 oz	0.8		
Cheese, cottage, 2% fat	1 oz	1.0		
Cheese, cream	1 oz	0.8		
Cheese, Edam	1 oz	0.3		
Cheese, goat, soft type	1 oz	0.3		
Cheese, Gouda	1 oz	0.6		
Cheese, Limburger	1 oz	0.1		
Cheese, Monterey	1 oz	0.2		
Cheese, mozzarella, skim milk	1 oz	0.8		
Cheese, mozzarella, whole milk	1 oz	0.6		
Cheese, Muenster	1 oz	0.3		
Cheese, Parmesan, grated	1 tbsp	0.2		
Cheese, Parmesan, hard	1 oz	0.8		
Cheese, Parmesan, shredded	1 tbsp	0.2		
Cheese, ricotta, part skim milk	1 oz	1.5		
Cheese, ricotta, whole milk	1 oz	0.9		
Cheese, romano	1 oz	1.1		
Cheese, Roquefort	1 oz	0.6		
Cheese, sauce	2 tbsp	2.0		
Cheese, sauce mix, prepared	1/2 cup	7.0		
Cheese spread, processed	1 oz	2.5		
Cheese, Swiss	1 oz	1.0		
Cherries, fresh, sour, red	1/2 cup	9.4		
Cherries, fresh, sweet, red	1/2 cup	12.0	22	3
Cherries, sour, red, light syrup	1/2 cup	24.3		
Cherries, sour, red, heavy syrup	1/2 cup	29.8		
Cherry juice	8 fl oz	30.0		
Chervil, dried	1 tbsp	1.0		
Chestnuts, Chinese, raw	1 oz	9.6		

Food	Serving size	Carb (gms)	GI	GL
Chestnuts, Chinese, dried	1 oz	22.7		
Chestnuts, European, roasted	1 cup	75.8		
Chestnuts, Japanese, dried	1 oz	23.1		
Chestnuts, Japanese, raw	1 oz	9.8		
Chestnuts, Japanese, roasted	1 oz	12.6		
Chicken	—	0.0	0	
Chicken gravy, canned	1/4 cup	3.0		
Chicken, lunch meat	1 oz	1.0	0	0
Chicken nuggets	6 nuggets	14.7	46	7
Chickpeas, dry, boiled	1/2 cup	22.5	32	7
Chicory greens, raw, chopped	1 cup	9.0		
Chicory roots, raw	1 root	10.8		
Chili, canned with beans	1 cup	30.0		
Chili powder	1 tbsp	4.4		
Chives, fresh or freeze dried	1 tbsp	0.1	0	0
Chocolate, bar, unsweetened	1 oz	8.0		
Chocolate beverage mix, powder	3 lg tsp	19.8		
Chocolate chips	1/2 oz	10.0		
Chocolate milk	1 cup	25.9		
Chocolate syrup	2 tbsp	24.8		
Cilantro, raw	1/4 cup	0.4		
Cinnamon, ground	1 tbsp	5.6		
Citrus fruit juice drink	8 fl oz	28.4		
Clam, boiled or steamed	9 large	5.8		
Clam chowder, see "Soup"				
Cloves, ground	1 tsp	1.4		
Club Soda	10 fl oz	0.0	0	0
Cocoa, baking, unsweetened	1 tbsp	3.0		
Cocoa mix	1 envelope	24.4		
Coconut meat, fresh, shredded	1 cup	12.0		

Food	Serving size	Carb (gms)	GI	GL
Coconut, flaked, sweetened	1 cup	10.5		
Coconut milk, canned	1 tbsp	0.4		
Cod	—	0.0	0	
Coffee, brewed	6 fl oz	0.8		
Coffee, instant, regular, powder	1 tsp	0.4		
Coffee, w/sugar, cappuccino	2 tsp round	10.5		
Coleslaw	1/2 cup	4.0		
Collards, fresh, boiled	1/2 cup	4.1		
Collards, fresh, raw	1/2 cup	1.2		
Collards, frozen, chopped	1/2 cup	6.1		
Cookie, animal crackers	1 oz	21.0		
Cookie, arrowroot biscuits	1 oz	17.7	63	11
Cookie, chocolate chip	1 oz	18.9		
Cookie, chocolate, cream filled	1 oz	19.9	64	13
Cookie, chocolate wafers	1 oz	20.5		
Cookie, digestive biscuits	1 oz	17.7	59	10
Cookie, fig newtons	2 pieces	20.0		
Cookie, fortune	1 oz	23.8		
Cookie, fudge	1 oz	22.2		
Cookie, gingersnaps	1 oz	21.8		
Cookie, graham wafers	1 oz	21.8	74	16
Cookie, marshmallow chocolate	1 oz	17.0		
Cookie, oatmeal, fat-free	1 oz	22.2	54	12
Cookie, peanut butter	1 oz	16.7		
Cookie, raisin, soft	1 oz	19.3		
Cookie, shortbread	1 oz	19.0		
Cookie, sugar	1 oz	19.2		
Cookie, vanilla, cream-filled	1 oz	20.4	77	16
Coriander, fresh	1/4 cup	0.1		
Coriander, dried, leaf	1 tsp	0.3		

Food	Serving size	Carb (gms)	GI	GL
Coriander, dried, seed	1 tsp	0.9		
Corn, canned, cream style	1/2 cup	23.2		
Corn, canned, kernel	1/2 cup	15.2	59	9
Corn, fresh, boiled, kernel	1/2 cup	20.6	59	12
Corn, frozen, kernel	1/2 cup	18.3		
Corn, on the cob, boiled	8 oz ear	29.4		
Corn chips, cheese curls	1 oz	16.0		
Corn chips, tortilla chips	1 oz	19.0	73	14
Corn flour (or Cornmeal)	1/4 cup	22.5		
Corn grits, cooked	1/2 cup	15.7		
Corn relish	1 tbsp	5.0		
Corn syrup	2 tbsp	30.0		
Corned beef loaf, jellied	1 slice	0.0	0	0
Cornstarch	1 tbsp	7.0		
Crab, Alaska king	—	0	0	
Crab, Alaska king, surimi	3 oz	8.5		
Crab, blue	—	0.0	0	
Crab, canned	—	0.0	0	
Crab, Dungeness, boiled	3 oz	0.8		
Crabapples, fresh, with peels	1/2 cup	11.0		
Cracker, cheese	1/2 oz	8.3		
Cracker, crispbread, rye	1/2 oz	11.6	69	8
Cracker, melba toast	1/2 oz	10.9		
Cracker, puffed rice cakes	1 oz	18.5	61	11
Cracker, rye wafers	1/2 oz	11.4		
Cracker, saltines	1/2 oz	10.2	74	8
Cracker, saltines, fat-free	1/2 oz	12.0		
Cracker, snack type	1/2 oz	8.7		
Cranberry, fresh, chopped	1/2 cup	7.1		
Cranberry juice cocktail	8 fl oz	35.4	56	20

Food	Serving size	Carb (gms)	GI	GL
Cranberry sauce, sweetened	1/2 cup	54.0		
Crayfish	—	0.0	0	
Cream, half and half	1 tbsp	0.6		
Cream, sour, non-fat	2 tbsp	4.0		
Cream, sour, regular	2 tbsp	1.0		
Cream, whipping	1 tbsp	0.4		
Cream soda	8 fl oz	32.0		
Cream substitute, powdered	1 tsp	4.1		
Creamer, non-dairy	1 tsp	1.1		
Creme De Menthe, 72 proof	1 fl oz	14.3		
Croissant, plain, buttered	2 oz piece	26.1	67	17
Croutons, plain	1/2 cup	11.0		
Cucumber, peeled, raw	8 1/4" long	8.3		
Cucumber, sliced	1/2 cup	1.6		
Cumin seed, ground	1 tsp	0.9		
Currants, European, black, raw	1/2 cup	8.4		
Currants, red or white, raw	1/2 cup	7.8		
Currants, Zante, dried	1/2 cup	53.3		
Curry powder	1 tsp	1.2		
Custard, mix, with milk and egg	1/2 cup	23.4		
Dandelion greens, raw	1 cup	5.0		
Danish cheese	2.5 oz piece	26.4		
Danish cinnamon	2.5 oz piece	31.0		
Danish fruit	2.5 oz piece	33.9		
Date, domestic, natural, pitted	10 dates	61.0		
Dill seed	1 tsp	1.2		
Donut, cake type	1 medium	18.8	76	14
Donut, chocolate, frosted	1 medium	20.6		
Donut, chocolate, glazed	1 medium	24.1		
Donut, cruller, glazed	1 medium	24.4		

Food	Serving size	Carb (gms)	GI	GL
Donut, jelly filled	1 medium	33.2		
Duck	—	0.0	0	
Egg, raw, white only	1 large	0.3		
Egg, raw, whole	1 large	0.6		
Egg, raw, yolk only	1 large	0.3		
Egg, hard-boiled, chopped	1 cup	1.4		
Egg, substitute	1/4 cup	1.0		
Eggroll	7" sq piece	18.5		
Eggnog, non-alcoholic	1 cup	35.6		
Eggplant, boiled	1 cup	6.5		
Eggplant, raw, with peel	1 cup	4.9		
Elderberries, raw	1/2 cup	13.2		
Enchilada Sauce	1/4 cup	3.0		
Endive, raw, chopped	1/2 cup	0.8		
Fat, any animal	—	0.0	0	
Fennel, bulb, raw	1 bulb	17.1		
Fig, canned, in heavy syrup	1/2 cup	29.7		
Fig, dried	5 figs	61.1	61	37
Fig, fresh	1 medium	9.6		
Filberts or hazelnuts, roasted	1 oz	5.0		
Fish, breaded, frozen	1 oz stick	6.7	38	3
Fish oil, any type	—	0.0	0	
Flatfish (flounder and sole)	—	0.0	0	
Frankfurter, beef	1 link	0.9		
Frankfurter, beef and pork	1 link	1.4		
French beans, dried, boiled	1/2 cup	20.7		
French toast, frozen	2.1 oz pce	19.0		
Frosting, chocolate	2 tbsp	24.0		
Fruit cocktail, canned, juice	1/2 cup	14.7		
Fruit cocktail, heavy syrup	1/2 cup	24.2	55	13

Food	Serving size	Carb (gms)	GI	GL
Fruit cocktail, light syrup	1/2 cup	18.8		
Fruit punch drink, diluted	1 oz	18.2		
Fruit salad, canned, heavy syrup	1/2 cup	29.8		
Garbanzo beans, dried, boiled	1/2 cup	22.5	32	7
Garlic	1 clove	1.0		
Garlic powder	1 tsp	2.3		
Garlic salt	1 tsp	0.5		
Gatorade, orange	8 fl oz	17.0	89	15
Gelatin dessert mix	1/2 cup	18.9		
Gin and tonic	1 fl oz	2.1		
Ginger ale	8 fl oz	21.6		
Ginger, ground	1 tsp	1.2		
Ginger root, raw	1/4 cup	3.6		
Goose	—	0.0	0	
Gooseberries, raw	1 oz	7.6		
Gram dhal, India, steamed	1/2 cup	11.1	11	1
Granola bar, chocolate chip	1 oz	20.4		
Granola bar, peanut butter	1 oz	17.7		
Granola bar, plain	1 oz	19.1		
Granola bar, soft, peanut butter	1 oz	18.2		
Granola bar, soft, raisin	1 oz	18.8		
Grape, fresh, seedless	10 medium	8.9	43	4
Grape, fresh, slipskin	10 medium	4.1		
Grape drink, canned	8 fl oz	30.0		
Grape juice, canned or bottled	8 fl oz	38.0		
Grape soda	8 fl oz	27.2		
Grapefruit, raw, pink or red	1/2 medium	10.6	25	3
Grapefruit, raw, white	1/2 medium	10.2	25	3
Grapefruit juice, unsweetened	8 fl oz	22.2	48	11
Gravy, see specific listing				

Food	Serving size	Carb (gms)	GI	GL
Green beans, fresh, boiled	1/2 cup	4.9		
Green beans, fresh, raw	1/2 cup	3.9		
Green pepper, sweet	1 medium	4.8		
Grouper	—	0.0	0	
Haddock	—	0.0	0	
Halibut	—	0.0	0	
Ham	—	0.0	0	
Ham, lunch meat, minced	1 oz	0.5	0	0
Ham and cheese spread	1 tbsp	0.3	0	0
Hamburger bun	1.5 oz	22.0	61	13
Hamburger patty	—	0.0	0	
Hearts of palm, canned	1 cup	7.3		
Herring, fresh or canned	—	0.0	0	
Herring, Atlantic, pickled	4 oz	10.9		
Hollandaise sauce mix, dry	2 tbsp	2.0		
Honey	1 tbsp	17.3	73	13
Honeydew melon, cubed	1/2 cup	7.8		
Horseradish, prepared	1 tbsp	1.0		
Hot dog	—	0.0	0	
Hot chocolate	1 cup	22.9	51	12
Hubbard squash, baked, cubed	1/2 cup	11.0		
Hummus	2 tbsp	5.7	6	1
Ice cream, chocolate	1/2 cup	18.6	62	12
Ice cream, strawberry	1/2 cup	18.2	62	11
Ice cream, vanilla	1/2 cup	15.5	62	10
Ice milk, vanilla	1/2 cup	15.0		
Italian sausage, cooked, pork	1 link	1.7		
Italian seasoning	1 tsp	0.6		
Jalapeno dip	2 tbsp	3.0		
Jam and preserves, fruit	1 tbsp	12.9	51	7

Food	Serving size	Carb (gms)	GI	GL
Jelly, fruit	1 tbsp	13.5		
Ketchup	1 tbsp	4.1		
Kidney beans, red, canned	1/2 cup	20.1	52	11
Kiwi Fruit, fresh, raw	1 medium	11.4	52	6
Lamb	—	0.0	0	
Lard, pork	—	0.0	0	
Leek, boiled	1 leek	9.9		
Lemon	1 wedge	2.9		
Lemon, peeled	2" dia	5.4		
Lemon juice, fresh	1 tsp	0.4		
Lemon-lime soda	8 fl oz	24.8		
Lemon zest	1 tbsp	1.0		
Lemonade, diluted	8 fl oz	24.8		
Lentils, boiled	1/2 cup	19.9	29	6
Lettuce, Boston	2 leaves	0.4		
Lettuce, iceberg	1 leaf	0.4		
Lettuce, romaine	1 leaf	0.2		
Lima beans, boiled	1/2 cup	20.1	32	6
Lime, fresh	2" dia	7.4		
Lime juice, fresh	1 tsp	0.5		
Limeade, diluted	8 fl oz	27.2		
Ling cod	—	0.0	0	
Liqueur, 34 proof	1 fl oz	6.5		
Liqueur, 53 proof	1 fl oz	16.4		
Liver, beef, pan fried	4 oz	8.9		
Liverwurst, pork	1 oz	0.6		
Lobster	4 oz	1.5		
Loganberries, fresh	1/2 cup	10.9		
Luncheon meat, beef	1 oz	1.7		
Luncheon meat, pork	1 oz	0.6		

Food	Serving size	Carb (gms)	GI	GL
Lychee, raw, shelled	1 oz	4.7		
Macadamia nuts	1 oz	3.8		
Macaroni, elbow	1 cup	39.7		
Macaroni, small shells	1 cup	32.6		
Macaroni, spirals	1 cup	38.0		
Macaroni, vegetable	4 oz	30.2		
Mace, ground	1 tsp	0.9		
Mackerel, Atlantic	—	0.0	0	
Mahi mahi	—	0.0	0	
Mangoes, fresh, peeled	1/2 cup	14.0	55	8
Maple syrup	1/4 cup	52.9	54	29
Margarine, all types	—	0.0	0	
Marjoram, dried	1 tsp	0.3		
Marmalade, orange	1 tbsp	13.3		
Marshmallow, cream topping	1 fl oz	22.5		
Martini, prepared from recipe	1 fl oz	0.1		
Mayonnaise, cholesterol-free	1 tbsp	2.2		
Mayonnaise, real	1 tbsp	0.4		
Melon, cantaloupe, raw	1 cup	14.2		
Melon, honeydew, raw	1 cup	15.9		
Melon balls, mixed, frozen	1 cup	13.8		
Milk, buttermilk, cultured	1 cup	12.2		
Milk, chocolate, plain	1 cup	31.0	34	11
Milk, condensed, sweetened	1 tbsp	10.4		
Milk, dry, instant, packet	3.2 oz	35.5		
Milk, dry, non-fat, regular	1/4 cup	15.6		
Milk, dry, whole	1 oz	10.9		
Milk, evaporated, skim	1 tbsp	1.8		
Milk, evaporated, whole	1 tbsp	1.6		
Milk, goat	1 cup	9.8		

Food	Serving size	Carb (gms)	GI	GL
Milk, low-fat, 2% fat	1 cup	11.7	33	4
Milk, skim	1 cup	11.9	32	4
Milk, whole, 3.3% fat	1 cup	11.4	27	3
Milk shake, thick, chocolate	8 fl oz	47.2		
Milk shake, thick, vanilla	8 fl oz	40.0		
Milkfish	—	0.0	0	
Millet, steamed, India	1/2 cup	34.8	68	24
Mixed nuts, dry roasted	1 oz	7.2		
Mixed nuts, oil roasted	1 oz	6.1		
Molasses	1 tbsp	13.8		
Monkfish	—	0.0	0	
Muffin, apple	2 oz	24.5	44	11
Muffin, blueberry	2 oz	27.4	59	16
Muffin, bran	2 oz	20.9	60	13
Muffin, carrot	2 oz	27.7	62	17
Muffin, corn	2 oz	29.0	49	14
Muffin, English, plain	2 oz	28.2		
Muffin, English, wheat	2 oz	25.5		
Muffin, oat bran	2 oz	25.2	69	17
Muffin mix, blueberry	1.75 oz	24.4		
Muffin mix, corn	1.75 oz	24.8		
Muffin mix, wheat bran	1.75 oz	23.3		
Mulberry, raw	1/2 cup	7.0		
Mushrooms, cooked, pieces	1/2 cup	4.0		
Mushrooms, canned	1/2 cup	3.9		
Mushrooms, raw	1/2 cup	1.6		
Mushrooms, shiitake	1/2 cup	10.4		
Mushroom, shiitake, dried	4 medium	11.3		
Mushroom gravy, canned	1/4 cup	3.0		
Mussel, blue, cooked	3 oz	6.0		

Food	Serving size	Carb (gms)	GI	GL
Mussel, blue, raw	1 cup	6.0		
Mustard, powder	1 tsp	0.3		
Mustard, prepared	1 tsp	1.0		
Mustard greens, raw or boiled	1 cup	2.8		
Mustard seed, yellow	1 tsp	1.2		
Navy bean, boiled	1/2 cup	19.8	31	6
Nectarines, raw, medium	2 1/2" dia	16.0		
Noodle, Chinese, cellophane	2 oz	48.0		
Noodle, Chinese, chow mein	1/2 cup	13.0		
Noodle, egg, cooked	1 cup	39.7		
Noodle, Japanese, soba	1 cup	24.4		
Noodle, Japanese, somen	1 cup	48.5		
Nutmeg, ground	1 tsp	1.1		
Nuts, mixed, dry roasted	1 oz	7.2		
Nuts, mixed, oil roasted	1 oz	6.1		
Oat, rolled or oatmeal	1/2 cup	27.0		
Oat, rolled or oatmeal, cooked	1/2 cup	22.5		
Oat, whole grain	1/2 cup	51.7		
Oat bran, cooked	1/2 cup	12.5		
Oat bran, uncooked	1/2 cup	31.1		
Oil, any type	—	0	0	
Okra, fresh, boiled	1/2 cup	5.6		
Okra, raw	1 cup	8.0		
Olives, green, with pits	10 large	0.5		
Olives, ripe, Greek, with pits	10 medium	1.7		
Onion, dried, minced	1 tsp	1.9		
Onion, green, raw, chopped	1/2 cup	3.7		
Onion, raw, chopped	1 cup	6.9		
Onion powder	1 tsp	2.4		
Onion rings, breaded	2 rings	7.6		

Food	Serving size	Carb (gms)	GI	GL
Onion salt	1 tsp	0.4		
Orange, mandarin	2" dia	9.4		
Orange, navels	2" dia	16.3	43	7
Orange, Valencias	2" dia	14.4	43	6
Orange drink, canned or bottled	8 fl oz	32.0		
Orange juice, canned or bottled	8 fl oz	24.8		
Orange juice, fresh	8 fl oz	25.6	46	12
Orange juice, frozen, diluted	8 fl oz	26.5	57	15
Oregano, ground	1 tsp	0.5		
Oyster, Eastern, wild, cook dry	3 oz	4.0		
Oyster, Eastern, wild, cook moist	3 oz	6.6		
Oyster, Eastern, wild, raw	6 medium	3.3		
Oyster, Pacific, cook moist	3 oz	8.4		
Oyster, Pacific, raw	3 oz	4.2		
Pancake, frozen, plain	4" cake	15.7		
Pancake mix, buckwheat	4" cake	8.5		
Pancake mix, prepared, plain	4" cake	11.0		
Pancake mix, whole-wheat	4" cake	13.0		
Pancake Syrup	1 tbsp	15.1		
Papaya, peeled, cubed	1/2 cup	7.0	56	4
Paprika	1 tsp	1.3		
Parsley, dried	1 tbsp	0.6		
Parsley, fresh	10 sprigs	0.6		
Parsnip, boiled	1/2 cup	15.4	97	15
Passion fruit, purple, raw	1 medium	4.2		
Pasta, corn, cooked	1 cup	39.1	78	30
Pasta, fettucine, egg	1 cup	46.1	32	15
Pasta, linguine, thin, wheat	1 cup	46.1	48	22
Pasta, macaroni, plain	1 cup	44.3	45	20
Pasta, plain, cooked	1 cup	39.7	71	28

Food	Serving size	Carb (gms)	GI	GL
Pasta, ravioli, meat filled	1 cup	38.3	39	15
Pasta, rice, brown	1 cup	38.5	92	35
Pasta, spaghetti, white	1 cup	44.3	41	18
Pasta, spinach, cooked	1 cup	36.6		
Pasta, tortellini, cheese	1 cup	26.6	50	13
Pasta, whole wheat	1 cup	37.2		
Pasta sauce, marinara	1/2 cup	12.7		
Pasta sauce, with mushrooms	1/2 cup	10.3		
Pasta sauce, with onions	1/2 cup	12.1		
Pastrami, beef	1 oz	0.1	0	0
Pâté, chicken liver	1 tbsp	0.9		
Pâté, goose liver, smoked	1 tbsp	0.6		
Peach, canned, heavy syrup	1/2 cup	25.5	58	15
Peach, canned, juice	1/2 cup	14.3	30	4
Peach, canned, light syrup	1/2 cup	18.3	52	10
Peach, dried, sulfured	1/2 cup	49.1		
Peach, fresh	2 1/2" dia	9.7	28	3
Peach nectar, canned	8 fl oz	34.5		
Peanut, dry roasted	1 oz	6.0		
Peanut, honey roasted	1 oz	8.0		
Peanut, oil roasted	1 oz	5.3		
Peanut, unroasted	1 oz	4.5	14	1
Peanut butter, chunky	1 tbsp	3.4		
Peanut butter, smooth	1 tbsp	3.3		
Pear, Bartlett, fresh, with peel	1 medium	25.1	41	10
Pear, dried, sulfured	1/2 cup	62.7		
Pear, fresh sliced	1/2 cup	12.5	33	4
Pear, halves in heavy syrup	1/2 cup	24.4		
Pear, halves in juice	1/2 cup	16.0		
Pear, halves in light syrup	1/2 cup	19.0		

Food	Serving size	Carb (gms)	GI	GL
Peas, green or sweet, boiled	1/2 cup	12.5	48	6
Peas, green or sweet, canned	1/2 cup	10.7		
Peas, green or sweet, fresh, raw	1/2 cup	10.4		
Peas, green or sweet, frozen	1/2 cup	16.2	51	8
Peas, snow, frozen	1/2 cup	7.2		
Peas, snow, raw	1/2 cup	5.4		
Peas and carrots, canned	1/2 cup	10.9		
Peas and carrots, frozen, boiled	1/2 cup	8.1		
Peas and onions, canned	1/2 cup	5.1		
Peas and onions, frozen, boiled	1/2 cup	7.8		
Pecan, dried	1 oz	5.2		
Pecan, dry roasted	1 oz	6.2		
Pecan, oil roasted	1 oz	4.6		
Pepper, black, whole	1 tsp	1.9		
Pepper, black or white, ground	1 tsp	1.7		
Pepper, chili, green or red	1/2 cup	7.1		
Pepper, red or cayenne	1 tsp	1.0		
Pepper, sweet, green or red, raw	1 medium	4.8		
Pepper, sweet, yellow, raw	1 large	11.8		
Pepper sauce, hot	—	0.0	0	
Peppermint, fresh	2 tbsp	0.4		
Pepperoni, pork or beef	1 sausage	7.5		
Perch	—	0.0	0	
Persimmons, Japanese, raw	1 fruit	31.9		
Persimmons, native, raw	1 fruit	8.5		
Pheasant	—	0.0	0	
Picante Sauce (salsa)	2 tbsp	2.0		
Pickle, bread & butter	1 oz	6.0		
Pickle, cucumber, dill	3 3/4" long	2.7		
Pickle, cucumber, sour	3 3/4" long	0.8		

Food	Serving size	Carb (gms)	GI	GL
Pickle, cucumber, sweet	3" long	11.1		
Pickle relish, hamburger	1 tbsp	5.1		
Pickle relish, hot dog	1 tbsp	3.4		
Pickle relish, sweet	1 tbsp	5.2		
Pickling spice	1 tsp	1.2		
Pie, apple	1/8 of 9" pie	42.5		
Pie, blueberry	1/8 of 9" pie	43.7		
Pie, cherry	1/8 of 9" pie	49.8		
Pie, chocolate cream	1/8 of 9" pie	31.9		
Pie, coconut custard	1/8 of 9" pie	26.5		
Pie, lemon meringue	1/8 of 9" pie	44.9		
Pie, peach	1/8 of 9" pie	32.4		
Pie, pecan	1/8 of 9" pie	58.0		
Pie, pumpkin	1/8 of 9" pie	26.7		
Pie crust, frozen	9" shell	62.7		
Pie crust, mix, prepared	9" shell	80.7		
Pike, northern	—	0.0	0	
Pimento, canned	1 oz	1.0		
Pina colada, prepared	8 fl oz	69.6		
Pine nuts, pignolia, dried	1 oz	4.0		
Pine nuts, pinyon, dried	1 oz	5.4		
Pineapple, canned, heavy syrup	1/2 cup	25.8		
Pineapple, canned, light syrup	1/2 cup	16.9		
Pineapple, canned, juice	1/2 cup	19.6		
Pineapple, raw, diced	1/2 cup	9.3	66	6
Pineapple juice	8 fl oz	34.4	46	16
Pistachio nuts, dried, shelled	1 oz	7.1		
Pistachio nuts, dry roasted	1 oz	7.8		
Pizza, cheese	1 slice	34.6	60	21
Pizza, super supreme thin	1 slice	17	30	5

Food	Serving size	Carb (gms)	GI	GL
Pizza, vegetarian supreme thin	1 slice	23.6	49	12
Plums, canned, heavy syrup	1/2 cup	30.0		
Plums, canned, light syrup	1/2 cup	20.5		
Plums, canned, juice	1/2 cup	19.1		
Plums, Japanese	2" dia	8.6		
Plums, raw, pitted, sliced	1/2 cup	10.7	24	3
Polish sausage, pork	1 oz	0.6		
Pollock	—	0.0	0	
Pomegranates, raw	1 fruit	26.2		
Popcorn, air popped	1 cup	6.2	89	6
Popcorn, caramel coated	2 oz	45.7		
Popcorn, oil popped	1 cup	6.3		
Poppy seed	1 tbsp	2.2		
Pork	—	0.0	0	
Pork rind snack, barbecue	1 oz	0.5		
Pork rind snack, plain	1 oz	0.0	0	
Potato, baked in skin	1 medium	51.0	85	43
Potato, baked without skin	1/2 cup	13.2		
Potato, boiled	1/2 cup	27.2	54	15
Potato, french fried	10 strips	17.0	75	13
Potato, fried	4 oz	38.6		
Potato, hash brown	1/2 cup	21.9		
Potato, mashed with whole milk	1/2 cup	18.4	67	12
Potato, mashed, milk and butter	1/2 cup	17.5	67	12
Potato, mix, mashed	1/2 cup	15.8	83	13
Potato, sweet (see "Sweet potato")				
Potato chips	1 oz	14.7	54	8
Potato pancakes	1 6" pancake	22.0		
Poultry seasoning	1 tsp	0.9		
Pretzels	1 oz	22.0	83	18

Food	Serving size	Carb (gms)	GI	GL
Prunes, dried	1/2 cup	58.8		
Prunes, heavy syrup	5 medium	23.9		
Prune juice	8 fl oz	43.5		
Prunes, pitted	5 medium	19.5	29	6
Pudding, banana	5 oz	30.1		
Pudding, chocolate	5 oz	32.4		
Pudding, lemon	5 oz	35.6		
Pudding, rice	5 oz	31.3		
Pudding, tapioca	5 oz	27.5		
Pudding, vanilla	5 oz	29.8		
Puff pastry, frozen	1.4 oz shell	18.3		
Puffed rice cakes	1 oz	18.5	61	11
Pumpkin, mashed	1/2 cup	6.0	75	5
Pumpkin pie mix	1/2 cup	35.1		
Pumpkin pie spice	1 tsp	1.2		
Quail	—	0.0	0	
Radicchio, raw	1/2 cup	0.8		
Radishes	10 medium	1.6		
Radishes, oriental	1/2 cup	1.8		
Radishes, white icicle	1/2 cup	1.3		
Raisins, golden	1/4 cup	28.9	64	18
Raisins, seedless	1/4 cup	28.7	64	18
Ranch dip	2 tbsp	3.0		
Raspberries, fresh	1/2 cup	7.1		
Raspberries, frozen, sweetened	1/2 cup	32.7		
Red snapper	—	0.0	0	
Refried beans, canned	1/2 cup	23.3		
Rhubarb, cooked, with sugar	1 cup	74.4		
Rhubarb, frozen	1 cup	6.8		
Rhubarb, unsweetened, raw	1/2 cup	2.8		

Food	Serving size	Carb (gms)	GI	GL
Rice, brown, long grain	1/2 cup	22.5	55	12
Rice, instant	1/2 cup	17.4	87	15
Rice, risotto	1/2 cup	25.5	69	18
Rice, white	1/2 cup	22.3	58	13
Rice, white, long grain	1/2 cup	22.3	41	9
Rice bran	1 cup	13.9		
Rice flour, brown	1/2 cup	60.4		
Rice flour, white	1/2 cup	63.3		
Rice mix, with pasta	1/2 cup	21.7		
Roll, dinner	1 oz	14.3	73	10
Roll, rye	1 oz	15.1		
Roll, wheat	1 oz	13.0		
Roll, French	1.3 oz	19.1		
Roll, hamburger, or hotdog	1.5 oz	21.6	61	13
Roll, kaiser	2 oz	30.1	73	23
Root Beer	8 fl oz	27.2		
Rosemary, dried	1 tsp	0.7		
Rutabaga, boiled	1/2 cup	7.4	72	5
Rutabaga, raw, cubed	1/2 cup	5.6		
Safflower seed, kernels	1 oz	9.5		
Safflower seed, meal	1 oz	13.7		
Saffron	1 tsp	0.5		
Sage, ground	1 tsp	0.4		
Salad dressing, 1000 Island	2 tbsp	4.8		
Salad dressing, blue cheese	2 tbsp	2.2		
Salad dressing, caesar	2 tbsp	2.0		
Salad dressing, French	2 tbsp	5.4		
Salad dressing, Italian	2 tbsp	3.0		
Salad dressing, Russian, low cal	2 tbsp	9.0		
Salad dressing, sesame seed	2 tbsp	2.6		

Food	Serving size	Carb (gms)	GI	GL
Salami, beef	1 oz	0.7		
Salami, beef and pork	1 oz	0.6		
Salmon, fresh, canned, smoked	—	0.0	0	
Salsa	2 tbsp	2.0		
Salt, table	—	0.0		
Sandwich spread	1 tbsp	1.8		
Sandwich spread, meatless	1 tbsp	3.4		
Sardine, fresh or canned in oil	—	0.0	0	
Sauerkraut	1/2 cup	5.1		
Sausage, pork, cooked	1 link	0.1		
Sausage, pork and beef	1 link	0.8		
Savory, ground	1 tsp	1.0		
Scallop, meat only	2 lrg or 5 sm	0.6		
Scones, plain	1 medium	11.8	92	11
Screwdriver, from recipe	1 fl oz	2.7		
Sea bass	—	0.0	0	
Sesame flour	1 oz	10.0		
Sesame meal	1 oz	7.4		
Sesame seeds	1 oz	7.3		
Shad	—	0.0	0	
Shallots, fresh, chopped	1 tbsp	1.7		
Sherbet, orange	1/2 cup	29.2		
Sherbet bar, orange	2.75 fl oz	20.1		
Shortening, any type	—	0.0	0	
Shrimp, meat only, raw	4 oz	1.0		
Shrimp, canned, drained	1 cup	1.3		
Shrimp, imitation	4 oz	0.4		
Snapper	—	0.0	0	
Soft drinks, club soda	12 fl oz	0.0	0	0
Soft drinks, cola	12 fl oz	39.0	63	25

Food	Serving size	Carb (gms)	GI	GL
Soft drinks, cola, diet	12 fl oz	0.0	0	0
Soft drinks, ginger ale	12 fl oz	38.0		
Soft drinks, orange	12 fl oz	52.0	68	35
Soft drinks, root beer	12 fl oz	43.0		
Soft drinks, tonic	12 fl oz	36.0		
Sole	—	0.0	0	
Sorbet, raspberry	1/2 cup	30.0		
Soup, bean/bacon, canned	1 cup	22.8		
Soup, bean (black), canned	1 cup	19.8	64	13
Soup, bean/ham (chunky), canned	1 cup	27.1		
Soup, beef, canned	1 cup	19.6		
Soup, beef bouillon, canned	1 cup	1.0		
Soup, beef bouillon, mix	1 cup	1.9		
Soup, beef/chicken, broth	1 cup	0.1		
Soup, beef noodle, canned	1 cup	9.0		
Soup, beef noodle, mix	1 cup	6.0		
Soup, cauliflower, mix	1 cup	10.7		
Soup, cheese, canned	1 cup	10.5		
Soup, chicken bouillon, mix	1 cup	1.4		
Soup, chicken broth, canned	1 cup	0.9		
Soup, chicken (chunky), canned	1 cup	17.3		
Soup, chicken (cream of), mix	1 cup	13.4		
Soup, chicken dumpling, canned	1 cup	6.0		
Soup, chicken gumbo, canned	1 cup	8.4		
Soup, chicken noodle, canned	1 cup	8.4		
Soup, chicken noodle, mix	1 cup	7.4		
Soup, chicken rice, canned	1 cup	7.2		
Soup, chicken rice, mix	1 cup	9.3		
Soup, chicken vegetable, canned	1 cup	8.6		
Soup, chicken vegetable, mix	1 cup	7.8		

Food	Serving size	Carb (gms)	GI	GL
Soup, chili beef, canned	1 cup	21.5		
Soup, clam chowder, canned	1 cup	18.8		
Soup, crab, canned	1 cup	10.3		
Soup, green pea, canned	1 cup	9.6	66	6
Soup, leek, mix	1 cup	11.4		
Soup, lentil, canned	1 cup	12.9	44	6
Soup, lentil with ham, canned	1 cup	20.2		
Soup, minestrone, canned	1 cup	20.7		
Soup, mushroom, canned	1 cup	11.2		
Soup, onion, canned	1 cup	8.2		
Soup, oyster stew, canned	1 cup	9.8		
Soup, Scotch broth, canned	1 cup	9.5		
Soup, tomato, canned	1 cup	16.6	38	6
Soup, tomato noodle, canned	1 cup	21.2		
Soup, tomato rice, canned	1 cup	21.9		
Soup, turkey noodle, canned	1 cup	8.6		
Soup, vegetable, canned	1 cup	13.0		
Soup, vegetable beef, canned	1 cup	10.2		
Soup, vegetable beef, mix	1 cup	8.0		
Soup, vegetable (chunky), canned	1 cup	19.0		
Sour cream, regular	2 tbsp	1.0		
Sour cream, non-fat	2 tbsp	4.0		
Soy flour, defatted	1 cup	38.4		
Soy flour, full, fat roasted	1 cup	28.6		
Soy meal, defatted, raw	1 cup	49.0		
Soy milk	8 fl oz	4.3	44	2
Soy protein, concentrate	1 oz	8.8		
Soy sauce, tamari	1 tbsp	1.0		
Soybean, dried, boiled	1/2 cup	8.5	15	1
Soybean, green	1/2 cup	14.1		

Food	Serving size	Carb (gms)	GI	GL
Soybean, green, boiled	1/2 cup	10.0		
Soybean, roasted	1/2 cup	28.9		
Spaghetti squash	1/2 cup	5.0		
Spareribs	—	0.0		
Spinach, boiled	1/2 cup	3.4		
Spinach, fresh	1/2 cup	1.0		
Spinach, frozen	1/2 cup	5.1		
Split peas, boiled	1/2 cup	20.7	32	7
Squash, summer	1/2 cup	2.3		
Strawberry, fresh	1/2 cup	5.2	40	2
Strawberry, frozen	1/2 cup	6.8		
Strawberry, heavy syrup	1/2 cup	29.9		
Strawberry drink mix	1 oz	28.1		
Stuffing, corn bread	1 oz	21.8		
Stuffing, mix	1 oz	21.6		
Sturgeon	—	0.0		
Succotash, cream corn	1/2 cup	23.4		
Succotash, frozen	1/2 cup	17.0		
Succotash, whole kernel	1/2 cup	17.9		
Sugar, beet or cane	1 tbsp	12.0	100	12
Sugar, maple	1 oz	25.5	100	26
Sugar substitute	1 packet	1.0		
Sunflower seed, dry roasted	1 oz	6.8		
Sunflower seed, kernels	1 oz	5.3		
Sunflower seed, oil roasted	1 oz	4.2		
Sunflower seed, toasted	1 oz	5.9		
Sushi, salmon	1 small	21.8	48	11
Sweet potato, baked	1 medium	27.7		
Sweet potato, boiled	4 oz	27.5	54	15
Sweet potato, mashed	1/2 cup	24.3		

Food	Serving size	Carb (gms)	GI	GL
Sweet and sour sauce	1 tbsp	7.0		
Swiss chard, boiled	1/2 cup	3.6		
Swiss chard, raw	1/2 cup	0.7		
Swordfish	—	0.0	0	
Taco shell	1 average	6.3	68	4
Tangerine, fresh	1 medium	9.4		
Tangerine, juice	1/2 cup	11.9		
Tangerine, light syrup	1/2 cup	20.4		
Tapioca, dry, pearl	1 oz	25.1		
Tarragon, ground	1 tsp	0.8		
Tartar sauce	2 tbsp	1.0		
Tea, regular or herbal	—	0.0	0	
Thyme, ground	1 tsp	0.9		
Tofu, fresh	1/2 cup	2.3		
Tofu, okara	1/2 cup	5.4		
Tom Collins, from recipe	1 fl oz	0.3		
Tomato, canned, whole	1/2 cup	5.2		
Tomato, dried	1/2 cup	15.1		
Tomato, fresh, boiled	1/2 cup	7.0		
Tomato, fresh, raw	1 medium	5.7		
Tomato juice	8 fl oz	10.0	38	4
Tomato paste	1 tbsp	3.0		
Tomato puree	1/4 cup	6.0		
Tomato sauce	1/2 cup	8.8		
Tomato sauce, with onions	1/2 cup	12.1		
Tonic water	8 fl oz	21.6		
Tortilla, corn, Mexican	1 average	20.7	52	11
Trail mix	1 oz	12.7		
Trout	—	0.0	0	
Tuna	—	0.0	0	

Food	Serving size	Carb (gms)	GI	GL
Turkey	—	0.0	0	
Turkey gravy, canned	1/4 cup	3.5		
Turmeric, ground	1 tsp	1.5		
Turnip, boiled, chopped	1/2 cup	3.8	72	3
Turnip, boiled, mashed	1/2 cup	5.6	72	4
Turnip greens, boiled	1/2 cup	3.1		
Turnip greens, raw	1/2 cup	1.6		
Vanilla extract, no alcohol	1 tsp	0.6		
Veal	—	0.0	0	
Vegetable juice, V8	8 fl oz	10.0	47	5
Vegetables, mixed, canned	1/2 cup	8.7		
Vegetables, mixed, frozen	1/2 cup	11.9		
Venison	—	0.0	0	
Vinegar	1 tbsp	1.0		
Waffle, buttermilk	4" square	13.5	76	10
Walnuts	1 oz	5.2		
Walnuts, black, dried	1 oz	3.4		
Water, bottled	—	0.0	0	
Water chestnuts, raw	4 medium	8.6		
Water chestnuts, fresh, sliced	1/2 cup	14.8		
Watercress	10 sprigs	0.3		
Watermelon	1 cup	11.0	72	8
Wheat, whole-grain	1/4 cup	34.2		
Wheat bran	2 tbsp	6.0		
Wheat flour, all purpose	1/4 cup	23.9		
Wheat flour, cake, white	1/4 cup	21.3		
Wheat flour, whole grain	1/4 cup	21.8		
Wheat germ	1 oz	14.7		
Whiskey sour, from recipe	1 fl oz	1.8		
White bean	1/2 cup	22.6		

Food	Serving size	Carb (gms)	GI	GL
Whitefish	—	0.0	0	
Wild rice, cooked	1/2 cup	17.5		
Wine, dessert or apertif	4 fl oz	9.2		
Wine, table or dry	4 fl oz	4.8		
Worcestershire sauce	1 tsp	1.0		
Yam, baked or boiled	1/2 cup	18.8	51	10
Yeast	1/4 oz pkg	2.7		
Yellow beans	1/2 cup	22.2		
Yogurt, chocolate	1/2 cup	17.9		
Yogurt, low-fat	8 fl oz	16.0	14	2
Yogurt, non-fat	8 fl oz	17.4		
Yogurt, plain	8 fl oz	10.6	36	4
Yogurt, vanilla	1/2 cup	17.4		
Zucchini, boiled, mashed	1/2 cup	7.8		
Zucchini, boiled, sliced	1/2 cup	3.5		
Zucchini, fresh	1/2 cup	1.9		

Fruits are listed from lowest to highest net carb content for easy reference. Nutrition information was calculated using the NutriBase Clinical Edition software. All whole fruits are medium sized. A serving size of ½ cup indicates that the fruit has been sliced, cubed, or diced.

Net Carbohydrate Content of Common Fruits

Fruit	Serving	Carbs	Fiber	Net Carbs
raspberries	1/2 cup	7.1	4.2	2.9
strawberries	1/2 cup	5.3	1.8	3.5
watermelon	1/2 cup	5.5	0.4	5.1
blackberries	1/2 cup	9.2	3.8	5.4
papaya	1/2 cup	6.9	1.3	5.6
peach	whole	8.8	1.6	7.2
honeydew melon	1/2 cup	8.1	0.5	7.6
plum	whole	8.6	1.0	7.6
grapefruit (pink)	1/2 fruit	9.2	1.4	7.9
blueberries	1/2 cup	10.2	2.0	8.2
pineapple	1/2 cup	9.6	0.9	8.7
tangerine	whole	11.0	2.3	8.7
kiwi	whole	11.3	2.6	8.7
orange	whole	15.4	3.1	12.3
mango	1/2 cup	14.0	1.5	12.5
grapes	1/2 cup	13.7	0.8	12.9
apple	whole	16.2	2.9	13.3
nectarine	whole	16.0	2.2	13.8
pear	whole	25.1	4.0	21.0
banana	whole	27.7	2.8	24.9

Raw vegetables are listed from lowest to highest net carb content for easy reference. Nutrition information was calculated using the NutriBase Clinical Edition software. A serving size of ½ cup indicates that the vegetable has been sliced, cubed, or diced. In cases where the fiber content is not listed, the software was unable to provide the information. Note the difference in fiber content between some raw versus cooked vegetables.

Net Carbohydrate Content of Common Vegetables: Raw

Vegetable	Serving	Carbs	Fiber	Net Carbs
avocado	1 ounce	0.5	0.6	0.0
romaine lettuce	1/2 cup	1.3	1.0	0.3
chinese cabbage	1/2 cup	0.8	0.4	0.4
broccoli	1/2 cup	1.9	1.1	0.8
leaf lettuce, red	1/2 cup	2.0	1.1	0.9
zucchini	1/2 cup	1.6	0.7	0.9
cauliflower	1/2 cup	2.0	1.0	1.0
bok choy	1/2 cup	1.0	0.0	1.0
leaf lettuce, green	1/2 cup	1.5	0.5	1.0
cucumber	1/2 cup	1.4	0.4	1.0
mushrooms	1/2 cup	1.4	0.4	1.0
savoy cabbage	1/2 cup	2.1	1.1	1.1
cabbage, green	1/2 cup	1.9	0.8	1.2
radish	1/2 cup	2.1	0.9	1.2
celery	1/2 cup	2.2	1.0	1.2
iceberg lettuce	1/2 cup	2.0	0.7	1.3
eggplant	1/2 cup	2.5	1.0	1.5
yellow tomato	1/2 cup	2.1	0.5	1.6
asparagus	1/2 cup	3.0	1.4	1.6
red pepper	1/2 cup	3.0	1.2	1.8
cabbage, red	1/2 cup	2.7	0.9	1.8

Vegetable	Serving	Carbs	Fiber	Net Carbs
green beans	1/2 cup	3.9	1.9	2.0
yellow beans	1/2 cup	3.9	1.9	2.0
brussel sprouts	1/2 cup	3.9	1.7	2.2
green onion	1/2 cup	3.7	1.3	2.4
tomato	1/2 cup	3.5	0.8	2.7
soybean sprouts	1/2 cup	3.4	0.4	3.0
pumpkin	1/2 cup	3.8	0.3	3.5
green pepper	1/2 cup	4.8	1.3	3.5
spaghetti squash	1/2 cup	3.5	0.0	3.5
bean sprouts	1/2 cup	3.8	0.0	3.8
red onion	1/2 cup	5.0	1.0	4.0
winter squash	1/2 cup	5.1	0.9	4.2
carrots	1/2 cup	6.2	1.8	4.4
hubbard squash	1/2 cup	5.1	0.0	5.1
onion	1/2 cup	6.9	1.4	5.5
acorn squash	1/2 cup	7.3	1.1	6.2
butternut squash	1/2 cup	8.2	0.0	8.2
sun-dried tomatoes	1/2 cup	12.8	3.2	9.6

Cooked vegetables are listed from lowest to highest net carb content for easy reference. Nutrition information was calculated using the NutriBase Clinical Edition software. A serving size of ½ cup indicates that the vegetable has been sliced, cubed, or diced. In cases where the fiber content is not listed, the software was unable to provide the information.

Net Carbohydrate Content of Common Vegetables: Cooked

Vegetable	Serving	Carbs	Fiber	Net Carbs
Chinese cabbage	1/2 cup	1.5	1.4	0.1
cauliflower	1/2 cup	2.6	1.7	0.9
cabbage, green	1/2 cup	3.4	1.7	1.7
broccoli	1/2 cup	4.0	2.3	1.7
celery	1/2 cup	3.0	1.2	1.8
asparagus	1/2 cup	3.8	1.9	1.9
cabbage, savoy	1/2 cup	4.0	2.0	2.0
cabbage, red	1/2 cup	3.5	1.5	2.0
eggplant	1/2 cup	3.3	1.2	2.1
zucchini	1/2 cup	3.5	1.3	2.2
mushrooms	1/2 cup	4.0	1.7	2.3
summer squash	1/2 cup	3.3	0.5	2.8
yellow beans	1/2 cup	5.0	2.1	2.9
green beans	1/2 cup	4.9	2.0	2.9
green pepper	1/2 cup	4.6	0.8	3.8
spaghetti squash	1/2 cup	5.0	1.1	3.9
pumpkin	1/2 cup	6.0	1.4	4.6
brussel sprouts	1/2 cup	6.8	2.0	4.8
red pepper	1/2 cup	6.2	1.1	5.1
carrots	1/2 cup	8.2	2.6	5.6
tomato	1/2 cup	7.0	1.3	5.6

Vegetable	Serving	Carbs	Fiber	Net Carbs
winter squash	1/2 cup	9.0	2.9	6.1
onion	1/2 cup	10.7	1.5	9.2
acorn squash	1/2 cup	14.9	4.5	10.4
butternut squash	1/2 cup	10.8	0.0	10.8
hubbard squash	1/2 cup	11.1	0.0	11.1
sweet potato, mashed	1/2 cup	24.3	3.0	21.3
sweet potato, baked	1 medium	27.7	3.4	24.3
potato, boiled	1 medium	27.4	2.7	24.7
potato, baked	1 medium	33.6	2.3	31.3
potato, microwaved	1 medium	36.3	2.5	33.8

Net Carbohydrate Content of Common Snack Foods

Snack Food	Serving	Carbs	Fiber	Net Carbs
cooked ham/ turkey/ beef/ chicken	1 oz	0.0	0.0	0.0
sugar-free Jell-O	1/2 cup	0.0	0.0	0.0
pork rinds	1/2 cup	0.0	0.0	0.0
Fresca or other diet drink	10 oz	0.0	0.0	0.0
herb tea	8 oz	0.0	0.0	0.0
cheddar cheese	1 oz	0.0	0.0	0.0
hard-boiled egg	1 egg	0.6	0.0	0.6
cream cheese	2 tbsp	0.8	0.0	0.8
cucumber	1/2 cup	1.4	0.4	1.0
celery stalk 8" long	2 stalks	3.0	1.4	1.6
ham and cheese Roll-Up	1 roll-up	1.8	0.1	1.7
Walnut Flax Muffin	1 muffin	3.2	1.1	2.1
Magic Muffins	1 muffin	7.6	5.1	2.5
almonds	1/4 cup	6.7	4.1	2.6
strawberries	1/2 cup	5.3	1.8	3.5
Flax & Oat Bread	1 slice	4.4	0.7	3.7
Oatmeal Flax Muffin	1 muffin	6.5	2.3	4.2
Walnut Pumpkin Loaf	1 slice	4.5	0.3	4.2
peanut butter	2 tbsp	6.2	1.9	4.3
Citrus Protein Bar	1 slice	5.4	1.0	4.4
Oatmeal Pumpkin Muffin	1 muffin	5.9	1.3	4.6
Coconut Zucchini Muffin	1 muffin	5.4	0.5	4.9
Orange Cranberry Muffin	1 muffin	7.5	2.6	4.9
peanuts	1/4 cup	7.9	2.9	5.0
Basic Bread	1 slice	5.1	0.0	5.1
Chocolate Nut Protein Bar	1 slice	7.3	0.9	6.4
plain yogurt	1/2 cup	7.0	0.0	7.0

Snack Food	Serving	Carbs	Fiber	Net Carbs
Flax & Oat Muffin	1 muffin	11.6	3.4	8.2
Lemon Carrot Muffin	1 muffin	10.4	1.4	9.0
cashews	1/4 cup	11.0	1.3	9.7
commercial low-carb protein bar*	1 bar	23.0	unknown	3.00

*Averge serving based on packaging information